I0199320

Optometry
in Mississippi

1920-2020

Optometry in Mississippi

1920 - 2020

moa

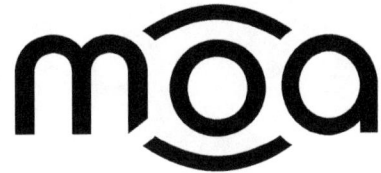

WILLIAM E. COCHRAN, O.D.

MISSISSIPPI OPTOMETRIC ASSOCIATION

Copyright 2021 by Mississippi Optometric Association

Author: Copyright 2021, William E. Cochran, O.D.
Editor: Copyright 2021, Peggy W. Jeans
Compiler: Copyright 2021, Linda Ross Aldy
Layout/Design: Copyright 2021, Hannah Lipking

All rights reserved

Published in the United States by the Mississippi Optometric Association, 141 Executive Drive, Suite 5, Madison, Mississippi 39110

The author and the publisher gratefully acknowledge the following source from which excerpts were used in chapter one:
American Optometric Association: A History 1898-1972 by James R. Gregg. Copyrighted 1972 by American Optometric Association. Excerpts used with permission of the American Optometric Association.

International Standard Book Number: 978-0-578-98115-4

Printed and bound in the United States of America

Library of Congress Control Number: 2021918614

Dedication

Optometry in Mississippi was significantly influenced by the leadership and dedication of Helen Allison St. Clair and Eric Muir, O.D. Their service, advocacy, and determination had a positive impact on the progress of the profession, and to its quality of vision and eye healthcare available to the citizens of Mississippi.

Thus, this publication is dedicated to the memory of the late Helen St. Clair, executive director, Mississippi Optometric Association, from 1976 until her retirement in 2005, and to the memory of the late Dr. Eric Muir, an active member of the Association from 1947 until his retirement in 2009.

6

Foreword

In 2020, the Mississippi Optometric Association celebrated the one-hundred-year anniversary of optometry as a legislated profession in Mississippi. While in Mississippi optometry began as a profession in the early 1900's, laws regulating the profession did not exist until 1920. This publication is a reflection of the history that has shaped optometry over the past 100 years.

The beginning of optometry as a profession in the United States in 1898 is documented in American Optometric Association, A History 1898-1972 by James R. Gregg, O.D., published by the AOA in 1972. Dr. Gregg's book details the association's early actions to establish optometry as a recognized healthcare profession across the country.

The passage of the Optometry Act in 1920 by the Mississippi Legislature created the Mississippi State Board of Examiners in Optometry. The Act was long sought by Mississippi optometrists. Since the beginning, members of the American and Mississippi associations have worked to improve optometric education, to advocate for the expansion of the scope of optometric practice, and to remain committed to serving the healthcare needs of the public.

This publication outlines the development of optometry in Mississippi. It aims to present an historical outline of how far the profession has evolved over the past century.

Acknowledgements

There are several people who participated in and supported the production of this historical text. The executive staff of Mississippi Optometric Association, Linda Ross Aldy and Sarah Link, deserve many thanks for coming up with the idea to tell the story of a century of optometry in Mississippi, and for their ongoing support.

Beverly Limbaugh, executive director, Mississippi State Board of Optometry, was instrumental in providing state board records without which this narrative would be incomplete. Thank you, Beverly.

L. B. Adkins, O.D., and his wife, Dixie, who attended all annual meetings and was active in the Women's Auxiliary, were helpful by relating their story in Mississippi Optometry.

Ed Muir, M.D., son of Eric Muir, O.D., is thanked for going out of his way to search for his dad's paper detailing the many legislative battles fought by optometry.

Contents

CHAPTER 01

In the Beginning

During the first year of optometry school, students learn of the very origin of optic science itself with the discovery of glass about 3000 B.C. Early on scientists recognized the limits in human eyesight. Galileo used his scientific knowledge of optics to develop the telescope.

Moreover, the word that gave the profession its name, optometer, first appeared in print in 1759 in A *Treatise on the Eye*, by William Porterfield, published in Edinburgh during the Age of Enlightenment. Porterfield wrote of an instrument he had "contrived for use in measuring the limits of distinct Vision, and in determining with great Exactness the Strength and Weakness of sight." He called it an *optometer*. A few years later, in 1784, Benjamin Franklin used his common sense to invent bifocals.

 "Between 1800 and 1890," according to Dr. Gregg,* "the skill of measuring the powers of human sight slowly developed, as well as the instruments necessary to make such an assessment. By 1890 the individuals providing these services were for the most part engaged in other businesses, usually jewelers. They did not call themselves optometrist but opticians or refracting opticians. However, the word optometry was used when referring to the determination of refractive errors."

In 1895, D. B. St. John Roosa, M.D., professor of ophthalmology and otology, New

American Optometric Association: A History 1898-1972 by James R. Gregg, O.D., is the primary source for information in this chapter.

York University, appealed to the members of the New York County Medical Society to "desist from giving support to non-medical men." Dr. Roosa called this an unethical practice, and at his urging, the Society adopted a resolution to expel any member who would send patients to opticians. Other state medical societies soon followed New York's lead.

Medical doctors began to fit glasses and threatened to pass laws to prevent anyone else from doing so. These incidents caused optometrists around the country to plan and organize in order to combat medical opposition. "Optometry deals with the public welfare," wrote Dr. Gregg, "and thus must be subject to some regulation to ensure the public that they will receive the finest visual care. Optometry as a profession, like other professions, must be regulated partly by legislative act, partly by self-control."

The New York Optometric Society introduced a bill as early as 1896 to regulate the practice of optometry, but was not successful until 1908. By then twelve states had passed legislation regulating the practice of optometry. Minnesota, in 1901, was the first state to do so, and North Dakota and California followed in 1903. The battle was on.

As early as 1895 an article in the *Optical Journal* called for the formation of a national organization 'to advance the science of optics and to promote the practice of Optometry.' Due to the growing opposition of medicine, a national organization was needed to lead a disciplined program to enact legislation regulating the practice of optometry.

"In October 1898 at the Broadway Central Hotel in New York City one-hundred-eighty-three charter members, representing thirty-one states and Canada, met to establish the American Association of Opticians (AAO). The delegates adopted a constitution and by-laws that stated, 'Any person engaged in the manufacture or sale of optical goods is eligible to active membership.' The membership included refracting and dispensing opticians, manufacturers, supply houses and importers."

Two years later in 1900 at the Detroit convention, at which three hundred members attended, membership in AAO was limited to refracting opticians due to the infighting of the various factions. During the meeting it was recommended that no one could become a member unless the practitioner was a graduate of a reputable optical school (no definition of reputable at this point) or a refracting optician in practice two years or more. There was a growing concern for the need of improvement in education.

"By the 1905 convention in Minneapolis at which 1,232 members attended, representing ten state affiliations, the American Association recognized the need to expand its role in passing legislation. There was a recommendation to provide sample bills for state associations, letters to guide optometrists in writing to legislators, and the ins and outs of lobbying. Raising the educational standards continued to be an issue."

At the 1907 annual convention in Kansas City, the following resolution was passed:

Whereas, The legitimate practice of optometry is being gradually encroached upon by unscrupulous and incompetent persons holding fraudulent diplomas issued by disreputable correspondence schools and the public wronged and injured by incompetent and unsatisfactory service and the profession injured, and

Whereas, Certain trade papers knowingly or unknowingly aid certain disreputable persons conducting such schools by publishing their advertisements:
Therefore, Be it resolved by the A.A.O. assembled in their tenth annual convention

at Kansas City, Mo. this day of the 25th of June, 1907, that we deplore this state of affairs and appeal to the legislatures of the several states to enact such legislation as shall put a stop to the method employed by disreputable schools, and that all optical trade papers stop advertising such schools, and that a copy of this resolution be sent to every state society of opticians and to all optical trade papers.

These were strong words, and the national association began to respond to false advertising. Soon there was a resolution calling for the establishment of a press committee to develop a public relations campaign for the new profession. In 1908, New York finally passed a law regulating the practice of optometry in an effort that had begun in 1896. It had been a bitter battle between the New York Optometric Association and the Medical Society of the State of New York. In a letter to New York legislators opposing the optometry bill, Frank Van Fleet, M.D., chair of the Medical Society opined, "To enact such a law will be to expose the people of the state to dangers which you can have no knowledge. To adapt lenses to the eyes of children without the use of the drug atropine, is little short of criminal."

Despite that, New York optometry prevailed, and it was a great triumph. With New York's success, eleven states soon followed in passing laws in 1909. During the 1908 convention in Philadelphia, Pennsylvania, the delegates addressed the issue of ethics and unanimously adopted the following code of ethics:

Code of Ethics off the American Association of Opticians

Each member should fully appreciate the responsibilities assumed by him and endeavor by unceasing study to qualify in the important work of ministering to the visual needs of his fellow men.

He should at all times emphasize the fact that optometry is a purely technical profession based upon a comprehensive knowledge of the mechanism of the human eye, the skillful manipulation of instruments for its adequate examination, and a knowledge of the properties of light and the relative effect thereon of lenses.

He should cultivate those sensibilities which permit the formation of standards for the generous appreciation of the work of others and the criticism of his own.

He should discourage the use of titles calculated to mislead or cause confusion in the public mind.

His methods of publicity should rigidly adhere to a dignified and modest statement of fact.

He should value his services commensurate with his ability, special preparation and skill, always welcoming the opportunity to be generous with his knowledge where it is needed, thereby realizing in fullest measure the true success which lies in the consciousness that the world has profited by his work.

It should be noted that throughout the early history of optometry practitioners were referred to in the masculine, "he," yet many female optometrists were in practice.

Up to this point, 1908, there had been great progress with thirteen states passing legislation regulating the practice of optometry. By 1909, eleven additional states had passed legislation. Now there were twenty-four state boards. This sudden growth in state boards created growing pains and issues arose -- state laws had to be enforced, examinations given, and licenses issued. There was a need for continuity across the nation.

"At the 1909 convention in Atlanta, Georgia, a group of state board members met to deal with the licensing issues facing the young profession. As a result, the National Board of State Examiners in Optometry was formed. Its purpose was 'to cooperate in unifying the examinations and provisions of the state laws.'"

In 1910, at the convention in Cedar Point, Ohio, the constitution was amended to change the name of the organization to the American Optical Association (AOA).

The 1913 convention was held in Rochester, New York. It was a popular meeting site due to the location of the headquarters of Bausch & Lomb and Eastman Kodak. Suppliers of optical instruments and equipment were located in Rochester as well, and they displayed the latest in eyewear and equipment at the convention.

During the education sessions, E.J. Brown, M.D. delivered a lecture on the pathology of the eye. "Strangely enough, four decades later official medicine would decide that it was unethical to teach optometrists how to detect disease," wrote Dr. Gregg. There was also growing interest in the business of optometry, or practice management, and the practical application of lenses. However, the lines between professionalism and commercialism were just beginning to be drawn.

At the San Francisco convention in 1915, education became the hot issue. There were no standards governing the various programs claiming to teach optometry. Some "schools" offered correspondence courses, and there were no standardized educational requirements. During the meeting, the National Organization of State Boards of Examiners in Optometry made specific recommendations for educational standards to the various states: "(1) 75% be the minimum standard on the written work on examinations; (2) the standard of clinical work be raised as high as practical; (3) all states require two years of high school {Yes, that is what you read!}; (4) the test book list of the AAO be used; and (5) the matter of reciprocity be studied."

It will be helpful to review a few of the schools considered "reputable" schools of optometry at the time. In 1872 George McFatrich founded a school in Chicago teaching refraction.

The Massachusetts College of Optometry was established in 1894; originally called the Klein School of Optics. In 1909, the school adopted the name Massachusetts College of Optometry, later becoming the New England College of Optometry.

In 1904, M.B. Ketchum, M.D., founded the Los Angeles School of Ophthalmology and Optometry. Subsequently, the word Ophthalmology was dropped and the name was changed to Southern California College of Optometry in 1972.
In 1907, the Needles Institute of Optometry was established in Kansas City, Missouri, and it merged with the Northern Illinois College of Optometry in 1926. In 1955, NICO merged with the Chicago College of Optometry to become Illinois College of Optometry.

In 1910, Columbia University in New York City became the first university to establish a stand-alone optometry program. The university closed the program in 1950.

In 1914, Ohio State University established a course in applied optics in the Department of Physics. This was a big deal as it was the first university to establish a degree in optics. In 1915, it became a four-year program, and the university designated it a separate college and began awarding the doctor of optometry degree in 1968.

"During 1915 and 1916 optometrists raised complaints that centered on nurses and school employees referring children with suspected visual problems to oculists (medical doctors) rather than to optometrists. Through public relations and printed materials developed by the AOA, many states ended this discrimination," Dr. Gregg wrote.

The following resolution was presented at the 1916 convention in Providence, Rhode Island:

That each member of (AOA) refrain from the words "free examination" in advertising -- passed.

Each state recommend passage of legislation requiring examination of all drivers of automobiles -- passed.

An assessment of $5 be levied on each member for securing legislation in states not having it -- failed.

That the name of the association be changed to the American Optometric Association -- referred to the next convention.

Shortly after the 1916 convention, the United States entered World War I. Many optometrists offered their services to the army and navy. However, the reply from the Surgeon General to P.A. Dilworth, chairman of the AOA Educational Committee, had indicated that only men with medical degrees could be commissioned and that regretfully his services could not be used. Thus, the status of the optometrist in the military service was purely a matter of chance.

In 1917, delegates to the American Optical Association Convention met in Columbus, Ohio. The main issue was the distinction between optometrists and the optical industry. The two groups met and agreed that a time be set apart at the AOA annual convention for a joint meeting of retailers, wholesalers, and manufacturers to discuss matters of business. There was a motion to rename the organization the American Optometric Association (AOA). Again the motion was tabled. A highlight of the convention was a visit by the delegates to Ohio State University's newly established program in applied optics. Faculty from the Physics Department presented many of the educational sessions.

During the 1918 convention in St. Paul, Minnesota, the major issue was professionalism versus commercialism. Does the optometrist provide a service or sell merchandise? Guest speaker Charles H. Mackintosh, an advertising specialist, spoke to the issue, "It will be difficult indeed for your profession ever to establish itself firmly in the public mind as a profession, while those among you who are most often in the public eye are so chiefly because of their merchandising ability." Mackintosh also called for the development of standards of practice and a fee-for-service system.

An important note is that the delegates passed a resolution favoring the women's suffrage movement. By the end of 1918, forty-four states had passed laws regulating the practice of optometry.

The 1919 congress in Rochester, New York, was attended by 1,290 delegates. A new constitution and bylaws were adopted and the name American Optometric Association was officially approved, wrote Dr. Gregg.

From the first meeting to form a national organization in 1898, the AOA slowly evolved into a cohesive organization representing the profession of optometry. There were many controversies along the way. The need for educational standards and public awareness programs became priorities. The success of the AOA was a result of the commitment and dedication of numerous leaders during this time of growth and development.

By the end of 1919, forty-six states had passed laws regulating the practice of optometry. In March 1920, Mississippi became the forty-seventh state.

CHAPTER 02

The Mississippi Optometric Association

The first meeting of the Mississippi Optical Society was held May 28, 1906. Its actions were recorded in the following article from the *Mississippi Optical Journal*, dated June 4, 1906:

"At the recent first meeting of this society (the Mississippi Optical Society), the organization of which is in the main the result of the efforts of W. E. Huston, the secretary of the American Association of Optometrists, the following were elected officers of the society for the coming year: E. R. von Seutter, Jackson, president; Theodore A. Marsh, Yazoo City; first vice-president; J. D. Crane, Gulfport, second vice-president; Albert A. Orr, Vicksburg, secretary; W. V. Waite, Corinth, treasurer. Executive Committee, J. D. Ellis, T. P. Martin, M. E. Fritz and A. L. Parker; Examining Committee, T. W. Queen, I. I. Guess and H. Watson."

From the *Mississippi Optical Journal*, dated November 1, 1906:

"This new society held a fall gathering at the Edwards House, Jackson, in October last. The meeting was spent discussing matters pertaining to the benefit of the influential organization. Among the regulations passed was the following, which will be of interest to the people of the State:

"Resolved; that all applicants for admission to this society be examined upon the following subjects: The anatomy of the eye, refraction, optics and practical experience.

"This society has had such a large growth that it feels the time (is) at hand when it can make admission into its membership a thorough test of the educational qualities of the applicant. Plans were also brought forth looking toward passing of a State law regulating the practice of optometry similar to that in force in California and Minnesota."

The next meeting of the Society was in June 1907 at the Hattiesburg Hotel. The attendees discussed a proposed optometry bill on the first day of the meeting, and approved an amended version the next day.

In 1909, the Society changed its name to the Mississippi Association of Optometrists.

Eleven years later the Mississippi Legislature finally passed the Optometry Practice Act, making Mississippi the forty-seventh state to enact an optometry law. License number 1 was issued to G. S. Sturm, Hazlehurst, on August 7, 1920. Over the next couple of days approximately one hundred and thirty-seven "optometrists" were licensed.

Unfortunately the early records and minutes of the Association have been lost to history; probably rotting away in an attic of a past secretary of the association. However, copies of the *Mississippi Optometrist*, beginning in 1948, and the Association minutes, beginning in 1958, have survived.

One can fill in those "lost" years by reviewing the records of the Mississippi State Board of Examiners in Optometry found in the next chapter. It also would be appropriate to surmise that the Association initiated some of the rules and regulations of the State Board. Moreover, it would not be hard to imagine the Association's activity at the time to be similar to that of the American Optometric Association, which were advocating for education, supporting ethical practice standards, and holding annual business meetings. We do know that the Women's Auxiliary to the Mississippi Optometric Association (note the Association's name change made in 1927) was organized during the 1935 annual convention held in Hattiesburg.

So what was going on in the life of optometrists during those "lost" years 1920 to 1950? Perhaps history can give some clues.

1920s

This decade is commonly referred to as the "Roaring Twenties." World War I had ended and a period of prosperity had begun. Women obtained the right to vote in 1920 through the Nineteenth Amendment to the U.S. Constitution, the League of Nations was established, and the Eighteenth Amendment to the U.S. Constitution prohibited the sale and distribution of alcohol. Some prices in the early 1920s were: a Ford Model T, $290; a typical house, $4,500; a pound of steak, 26 cents; a loaf of bread, 7 cents; a dozen eggs, 34 cents, and a quart of milk, 9 cents.

1930s

This decade was overshadowed by the Great Depression, which would last beyond ten years in Mississippi. It began with the October 1929 stock market crash. The collapsed economy resulted in unprecedented unemployment and widespread poverty. Franklin D. Roosevelt, elected U.S. President in 1933, implemented the New Deal legislation, a domestic program designed to bring jobs and economic relief across the country. Due to the financial crisis one can conclude that there was a drop in Association membership.

1940s

World War II dominated the early 1940s. The war effort brought about an explosion in the development of technology. The first programmable electronic digital computer, ENIAC, was developed at the University of Pennsylvania. At the end of the war in 1945, the Baby Boom began, as did a steady increase in inflation. In 1940, a typical new house cost $3,920, by 1949, $7,450, and the cost of a new car rose from $850 to $1,420. In recognition of their military service, veterans became eligible for financial and educational benefits in the GI Bill of Rights. As a result, veterans were able to pursue a college education, and many enrolled in optometry school. On December 31, 1947, the Mississippi Optometric Association was incorporated.

1950s

J. W. Rothchild, O.D., Oxford, was the first editor and publisher of the *Mississippi Optometrist*. Although it is not known when the first issue was published, it is known that Irvin Mauldin, O.D., Corinth, became the second editor and publisher in the latter part of 1948. In his first editorial Dr. Mauldin wrote, "To us as members of a young and growing profession, the year 1949 offers many responsibilities and opportunities. We have much to do in optometry. Let us be about that work!"

In January 1950, the Association passed a resolution adopting a code of ethics that barred "nonprofessional" optometrists from becoming members of the state Association. The association hired attorney Richard A. Billups Jr. as legal counsel. Prior to moving to Mississippi, Billups had been successful in aiding the Oklahoma Optometric Association in its effort to combat commercialism. Dr. Eric Muir's 1981 paper delivered at the Association's planning conference (see Appendix), described the struggle to enhance optometry's image by fighting its sometime blatant commercialism, and by encouraging continuing education.

To get an idea of the commercial issue, the American Optometric Association stated in the November 1950 issue of *Redbook* magazine: "Members of the American Optometric Association are pledged to conduct their practices along purely professional lines. Unfortunately, they have no jurisdiction over the neon lights and blatant advertising of the quickie eyeglass parlors."

Billups pointed out that a new law was not needed to combat commercialism; that the existing optometry law prohibited commercialism as it was the "unlawful practice of optometry." Consequently, in early 1951, an injunction was filed against Sears, Roebuck and Company seeking to enjoin them from the unlawful practice of optometry. Optometry won the lawsuit. The opinion of the court was: "The advent of the optometrist and the increasing need for his services in this competitive and complex age makes it of extreme importance that he measure up to all the requirements and serve his patrons to the best of his ability, and in the spirit and purpose of the law that approves him worthy of his profession and of the franchise granted him to practice it." In 1952, the Mississippi Supreme Court upheld the lower court's decision.

Throughout the 1950s, the Association's priorities included the recruitment of members, promoting continuing education, developing public relations programs, and responding to challenges of ophthalmology. To promote the importance of eye care, a Speaker's Bureau was initiated. The Mississippi State Board of Health approved changes in the administration policies of the Sight Conservation Program for school children that made optometrists eligible for payment for refraction and glasses on the same basis as ophthalmologists. The first African American optometrist licensed in Mississippi, Dr. David W. White, Jackson, took and passed the board exam at the Woolfolk Building on July 9, 1951. He remained the only African American optometrist in the state until 1978 when Dr. Linda D. Johnson and Dr. Robert E. Lee were licensed.

In January 1956, the annual education meeting was held at the University of Mississippi, or Ole Miss. Optometric meetings at Ole Miss were seriously contested by medicine. Two years later, the Mississippi State Medical Association proposed a resolution saying that optometry was a "cult" and requested that the university not allow optometric meetings nor its speakers on campus.

1960s

The bylaws of the Association were amended in 1963 to expand the number of board members from five to seven. The next year, the Association petitioned the State Board to adopt a regulation requiring twenty hours of post-graduate optometric study each year as a prerequisite for license renewal. The State Board adopted the regulation. Consequently, one hundred and eight optometrists registered for the 1965 Ole Miss Continuing Education Program. It was the largest attendance ever.

Also in 1965, Title XIX, the Medical Assistance Program (Medicaid), went into effect.

During the 1966 Mississippi legislative session, SB 1655, the freedom of choice bill was passed, which gave equal status for insurance claims to medical doctors and optometrists. The legislature also approved a bill providing for an optometrist to be on the Mississippi State Board of Health. Governor Paul Johnson Jr. appointed Dr. Eric Muir, Cleveland, to represent optometry on the board. Governor Johnson also proclaimed the week of March 17, 1966, as "Save Your Vision Week."

During the 1966 annual summer convention at the Buena Vista Hotel in Biloxi, a resolution was passed calling for the repeal of the American Medical Association's Resolution #77, which prohibited the recognition of optometry as a profession. During the meeting, it was announced that Medicare now approved post-operative cataract prosthetic services by optometrists (note: not examination).

Dr. Robert B. Griffin, Indianola, was named Mississippi's first *Optometrist of the Year* during the November 1967 business meeting.

During 1968, the Association's board decided not to support SB 217, which would license ophthalmic technicians, and adopted a resolution establishing a minimum fee of $25 for a comprehensive exam based on a relative point value system.

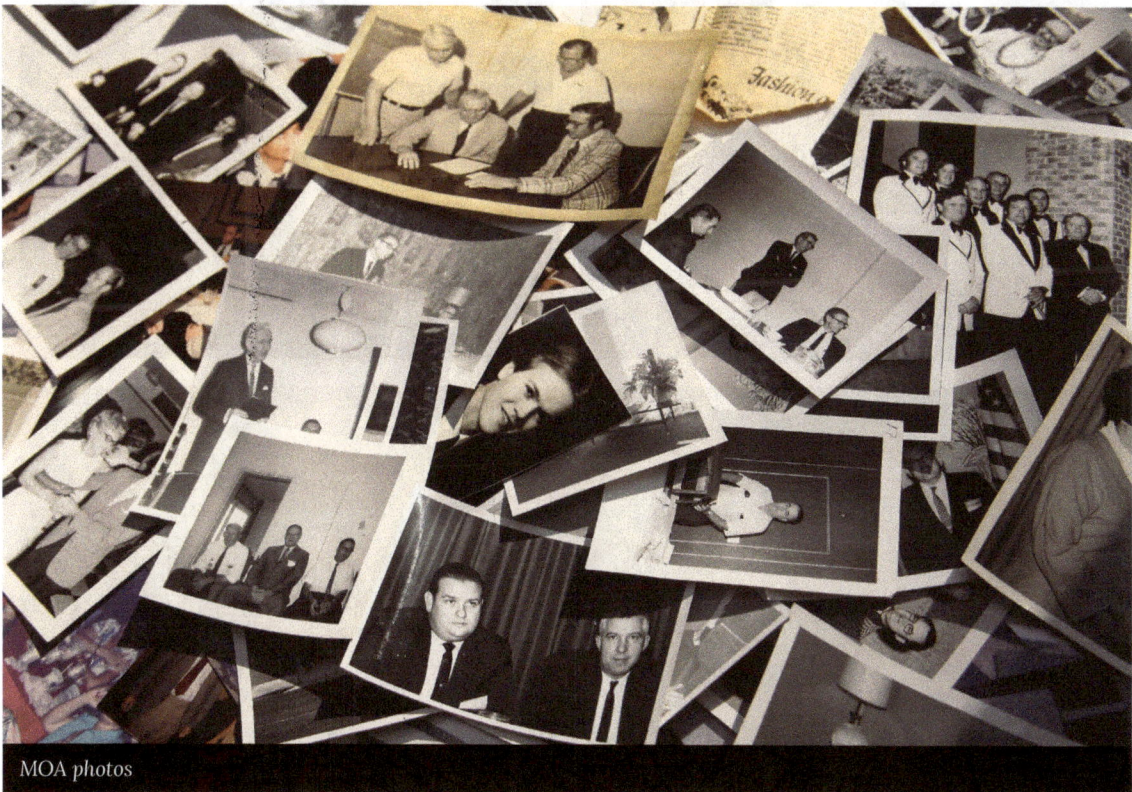

MOA photos

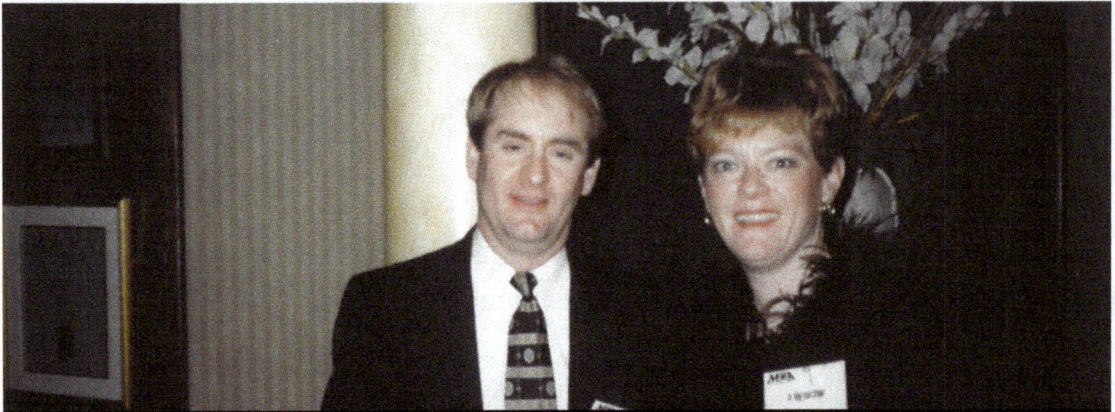

Todd Hall, OD and Amy Crigler, OD welcome guests.

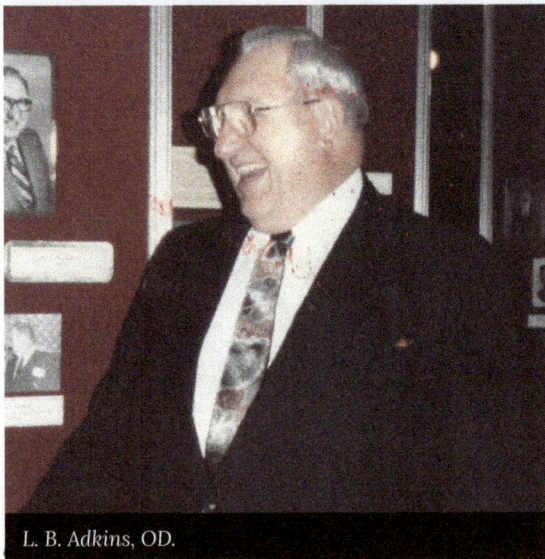

L. B. Adkins, OD.

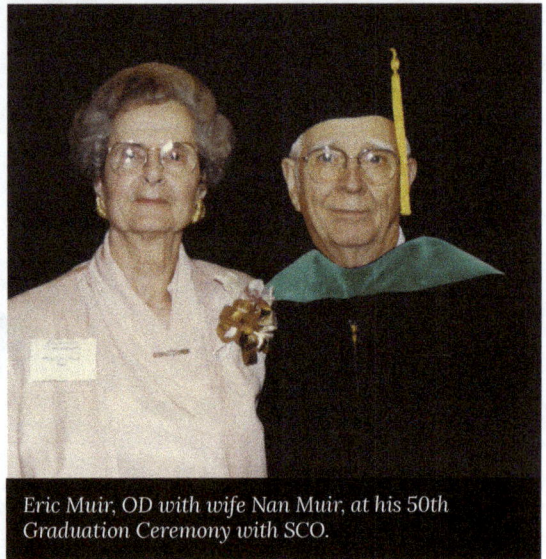

Eric Muir, OD with wife Nan Muir, at his 50th Graduation Ceremony with SCO.

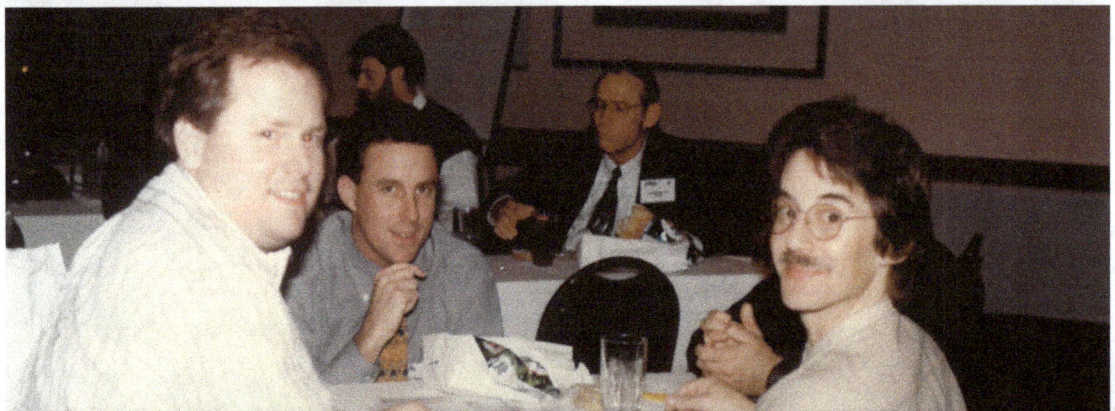

Background: Bernard Ellis, OD. L-R: Ty Hubbard, OD. David Parker, OD. Glenn Goldring, OD.

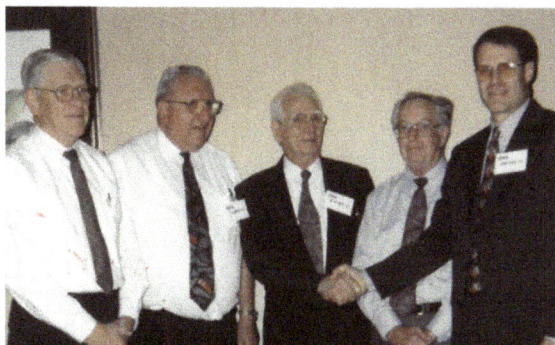

MOA 40th Annual Education Conference. L-R: Jim Wright OD, LB Adkins OD, Eric Muir OD, Carl Von Suetter OD, Frank Evans OD.

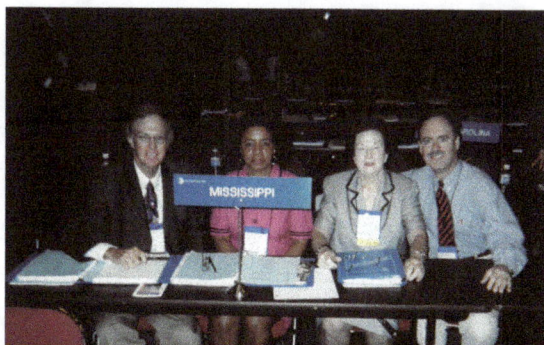

AOA House of Delegates. L-R: Wilburn "Bill" Lord OD, Linda Johnson OD, Helen St. Clair CAE, William Strickland, OD.

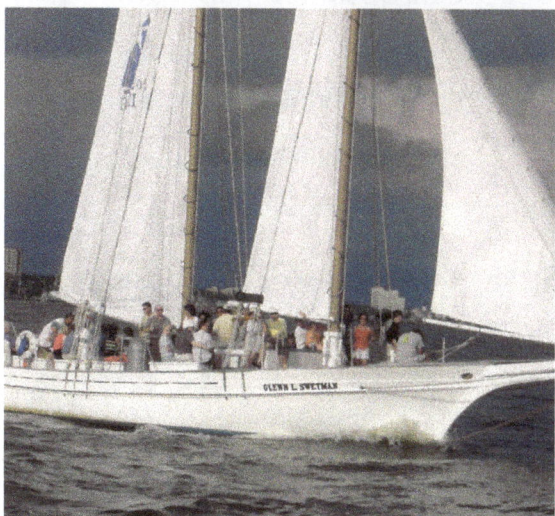

MOA Summer Convention event.

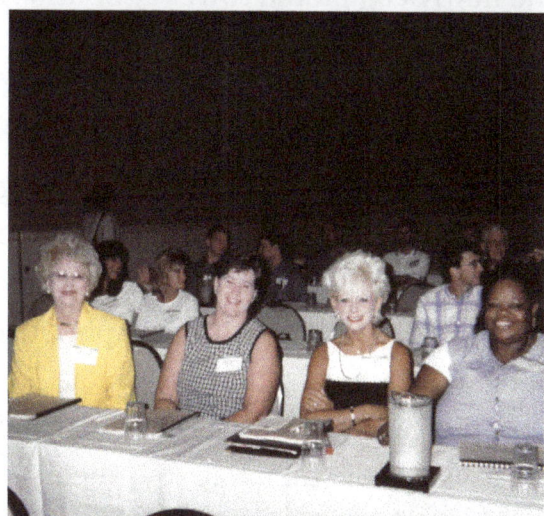

Mississippi Paraoptometrics.

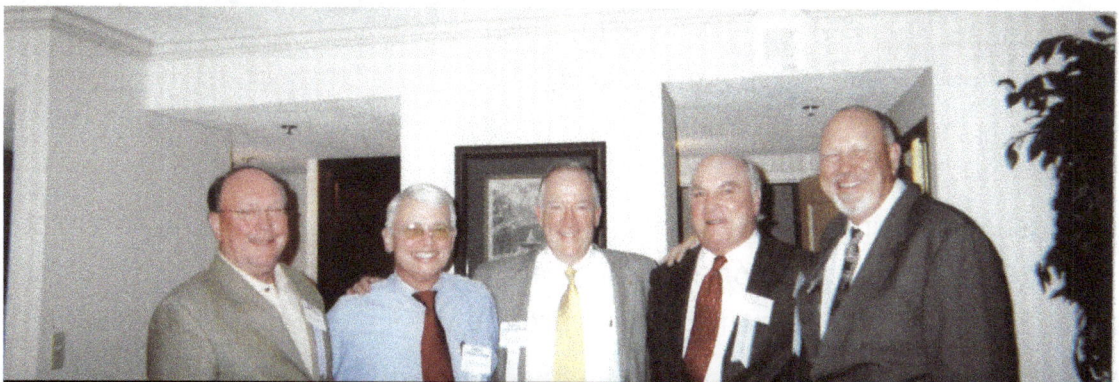

MOA Past President's reception. L-R: Watts Davis OD (Laurel), Earl Malone OD (Biloxi), Billy Cochran OD (Memphis, TN), Jerry Hollis OD (Jackson's Gap, AL), C. Lowell Jones OD (Indianola, MS).

1970s

This decade saw significant growth in membership from one hundred and five to one hundred and forty-three. The Association hired its first full-time executive director in 1973, and Helen St. Clair was named the second executive director in 1976. The Association lobbied consistently throughout the decade to expand the scope of practice. In 1970, Association dues were increased from $15 to $50 per year. The 1970 annual convention met in Memphis along with the Tennessee and Arkansas associations to participate in the dedication of the newly completed tower at Southern College of Optometry, or SCO.

Beginning in 1974, legislation was introduced authorizing optometrists the use of pharmaceutical agents for diagnostic purposes. To enhance the efforts to expand the scope of practice, the Association sponsored graduate courses in pharmacology presented by SCO and Pennsylvania College of Optometry. Yet these efforts were challenged every step of the way by medicine and ophthalmology. During the 1975 legislative session, ophthalmology testified that two of *their* patients had died, and that one hundred and seventeen had suffered cardiac arrest

Helen St. Clair, CAE

when diagnostic pharmaceutical agents were administered.

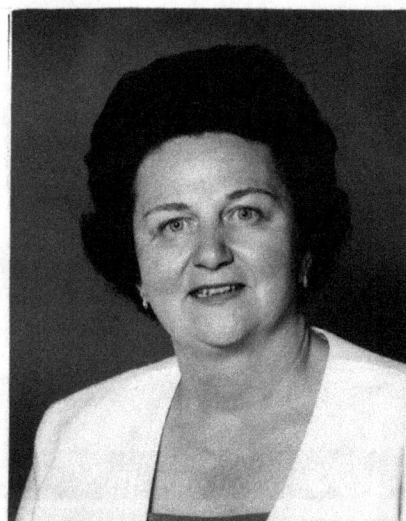

The Association sponsored several public relations programs to inform the public of the importance of eye safety and good vision. Mississippi led the nation in blindness at the time. These programs included national Save Your Vision Week, Seymour Safely, and the film *Dr. Tom and His Magic Tree*. In 1974, the Mississippi Optometric Political Action Committee was established.

The Mississippi Auxiliary was presented two first-place awards during the 1974 AOA convention in Washington, D.C., and in 1975, the auxiliary hosted the annual AOA Auxiliary breakfast in Hot Springs, Arkansas. In 1979, the auxiliary hosted the annual Southern Educational Congress of Optometry, or SECO, luncheon. The theme was "Mississippi Down Home." The state's optometric assistants formally organized in August 1975, and elected Joann Johnston as president.

Other noteworthy events during the 1970s included Southern Regional Educational Board's funding for optometry student scholarships, Dr. L.B. Adkins' election as president of SECO, and the first annual strategic planning retreat held at Lake Tiak-O'Khata. The Association's membership reached an all-time high in 1978 at one hundred and forty-nine.

The 1978 annual convention met in New Orleans in conjunction with the AOA's annual meeting, at which the AOA launched the National Consumer Communications Program designed to promote optometry through television, newspaper, and magazine publications. The program was supported by an assessment increase to AOA members of $100 per year for three years.

The Mississippi Optometric Association's attorney, Richard Billups Jr., retired after faithfully serving Mississippi optometry, and attorney Delbert Hosemann Jr. was appointed the Association's legal counsel. (Hosemann is now the 2020–2024 Lieutenant Governor of Mississippi.) The Federal Trade Commission mandated that spectacles and contact lens prescriptions be given to patients effective January 1979. The 1979-80 Association budget was $51,236. According to Association records, there was only one woman in active practice by 1970, Dr. Nell Edgar Niles, Kosciusko. That record changed shortly thereafter in the late 1970s with the addition of new members: Dr. Sallye Sawyer Scott, Senatobia; Dr. Linda Johnson, Jackson; Dr. Amy Ajax Crigler, Starkville; and Dr. Connie Long, Aberdeen. These pioneers set the standard for their future colleagues.

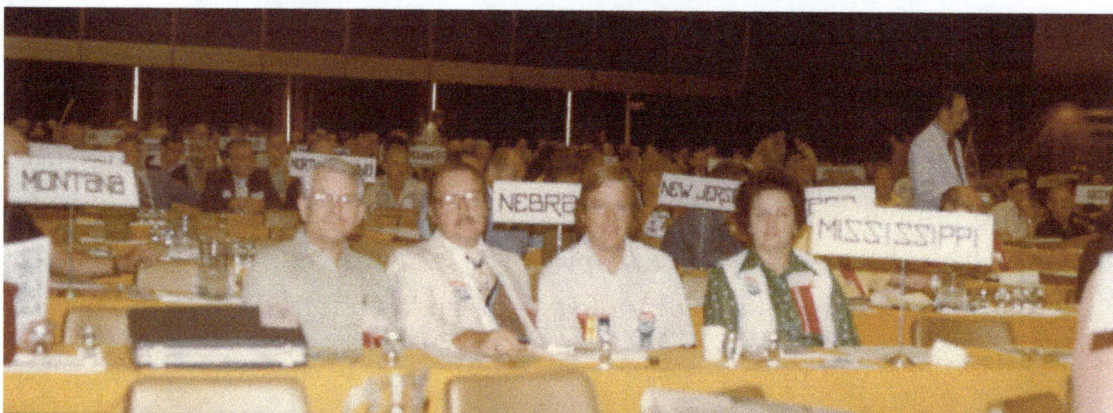

AOA House of Delegates.

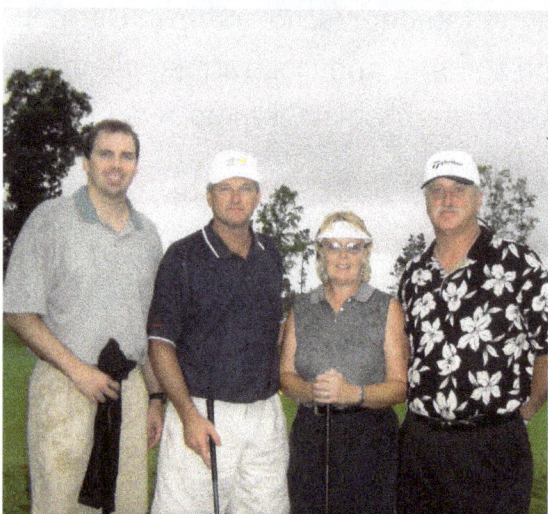

MOA Golf Outing at Summer Convention.

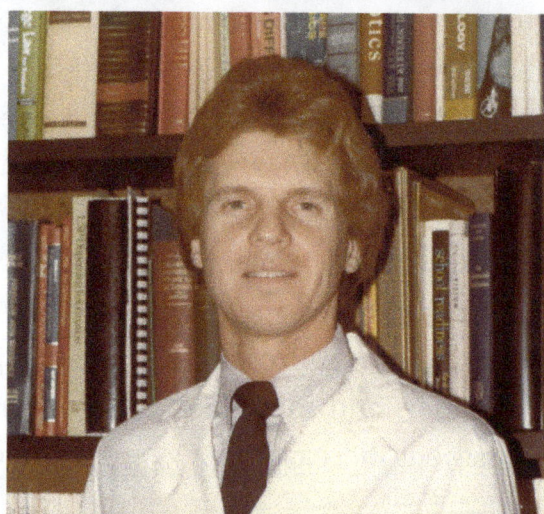

James P. Brownlee, OD

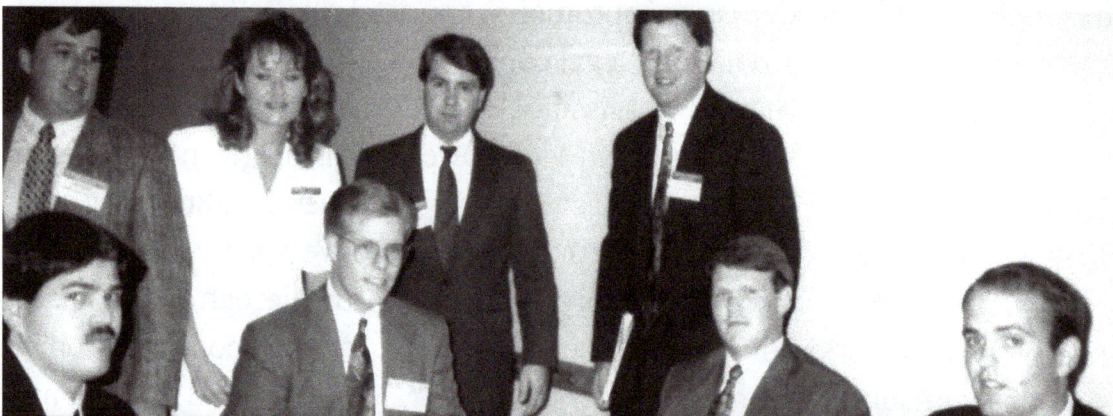

MOA hosts reception for new optometrists.

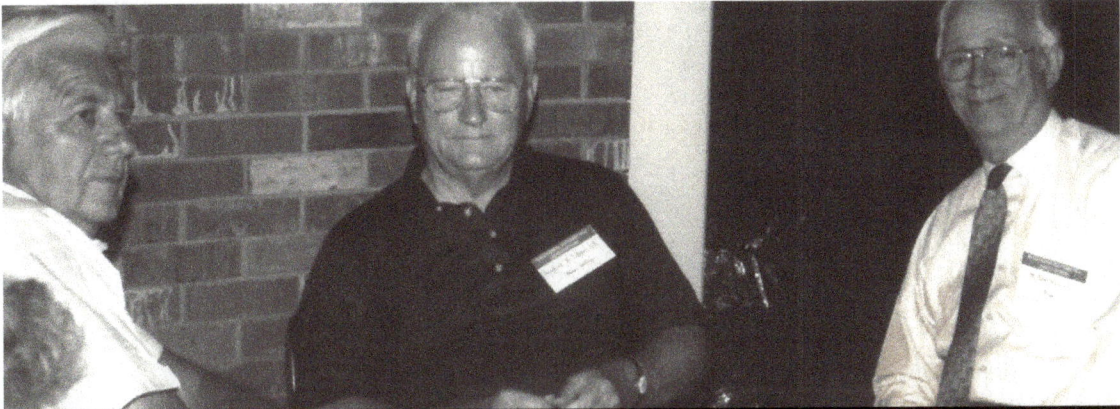

L-R: Horace May OD, Rayford Edgar OD, Eric Muir OD.

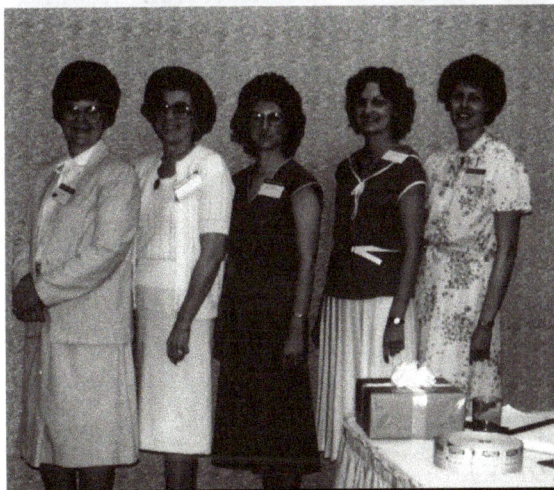

MOA Auxillary officers (this group later became the Mississippi Paraoptometric Association).

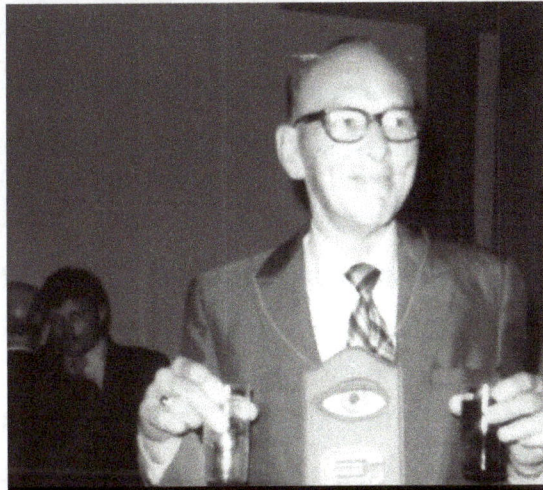

W.F. Clark, OD (Meridian). MOA's perennial court jester!

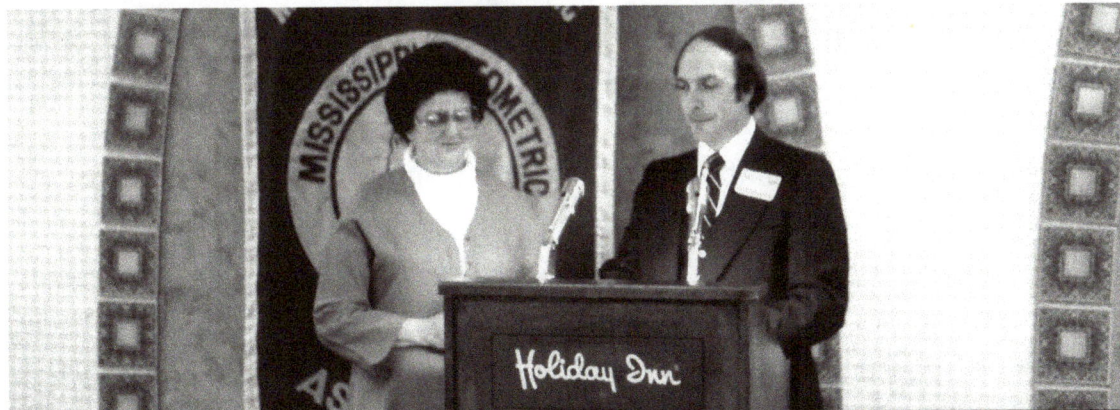

MOA Education Conference. Helen St. Clair and Watts Davis, OD.

1980s

The decade began with the Association's 1980 annual convention meeting in Hawaii.

The battle with ophthalmology intensified. Encouraged by the Physician's Eye Network (PEN), the Disabled American Veterans passed a resolution in 1980 to prohibit optometrists from administering primary eye care at Veterans Administration (VA) facilities. The PEN, a national quarterly newspaper organized by ophthalmology, opposed the profession of optometry. In the long run, the publication fizzled, and optometrists continued to provide service to the VA.

The attacks against optometry continued with ophthalmology urging the Mid-South Lion's Sight Service to pass a resolution which in effect accused the optometry profession of "offensive and diversive [sic]" actions in its attempt to update state laws to allow the public the benefit of contemporary optometry. Despite medicine's best efforts, HB 475 allowing the use of diagnostic pharmaceutical agents by optometrists passed, and was signed into law by Governor William Winter in April 1982. Mississippi became the thirty-second state to grant DPA privileges. This achievement was a result of an overwhelming number of Association members doing their "homework" under the direction of legislative chairman, Dr. Jim Brownlee, Laurel, and legislative advocate, Cliff Thomson.

Perhaps the most significant *national* event during the 1980s was the passage of federal legislation that optometry had consistently sought for two decades: Medicare parity. The legislation, effective April 1987, provided approval to "reimburse doctors of optometry for covered Medicare services within their state licensure." This victory was the result of years of lobbying Congress by the AOA and by every state association. The American Academy of Ophthalmology took issue with the newly enacted expansion of Medicare coverage extended to optometry. That same year, Governor Bill Allain, signed SB 2464 prohibiting anyone except a licensed optometrist or ophthalmologist from fitting contact lenses.

Throughout the decade, Association members received recognition for their accomplishments. Dr. Sallye S. Scott, Senatobia, became the first woman to be elected to the MOA Board. Dr. Jerry Hayes, Vicksburg, was named a consulting editor to *Optometric Management*. Joann Johnston, Hattiesburg, was named Optometric Assistant of the South. Dr. Larry Routt, Kosciusko, wrote an editorial published in the Journal of the AOA. Dr. Jim Herrington, Hattiesburg, and Dr. Bob Traylor, Clarksdale, served terms as president of the Southern Council of Optometry. Dr. Horace May, Newton, was named Mississippi's Optometrist of the Year. MOA's executive director, Helen St. Clair, received her designation as a Certified Association Executive (CAE). Dr. John White, Baldwyn, became the first Mississippi optometrist to be elected to the state Senate. Dr. Amy A. Crigler, Starkville, was selected as Mississippi's Outstanding Career Woman. Former MOA president, Dr. Billy Cochran, Kosciusko, was inaugurated as president of Southern College of Optometry, succeeding Dr. Spurgeon Eure, Hattiesburg, also a former MOA member.

The AOA House of Delegates named Dr. Connie Long, Aberdeen, the winner of the Optometric Recognition Award by having the most C.E. hours of any optometrist in the national ORA program.

There were many events of significance during the 1980s. The Federal Trade Commission proposed the "Eyeglass II" rule seeking to preempt state bans on the commercial practice of optometry. One hundred twenty-two Mississippi optometrists completed a nine-month TPA course. The annual education conference was moved from Ole Miss to Jackson for budgetary reasons. The Jackson Eye Institute, Mississippi's first co-management center, opened in Jackson. The first annual Vision Exposition was held in Jackson during the fall education conference. This event highlighted the many optical laboratories, frame companies, and ophthalmic suppliers supporting MOA. Mississippi hosted the National Optometric Association's annual meeting in Jackson. The NOA, founded in 1969 by twenty-five African Americans at a meeting in Virginia, has as its mission to deliver eye and vision care services to urban and minority communities.

The Association's beloved Richard A. Billups Jr., legal counsel to the State Board and to the Association for over thirty-five years, passed away. The Association retained a public relations firm to promote public awareness of the need for professional eye examinations and for hunter safety. The AOA's Practice Enhancement Program (PEP) was launched with the initial phase of the program designed to help the professional practitioner maintain quality patient care while meeting the challenges presented by mass merchandisers and ophthalmology. Dr. Jeff Minor, Flowood, served as the first state chairman of PEP.

1990s

The Association continued its efforts to expand the scope of practice in keeping with the education and training of doctors of optometry. In January 1990, a TPA bill was introduced in the House and the Senate to no avail. However, a TPA bill passed four years later and Governor Kirk Fordice signed it into law effective March 29, 1994. Mississippi became the thirty-eighth state to authorize the use of pharmaceutical agents for treatment purposes. Association president, Dr. Glen Stribling, Jackson, and legislative chairman, Dr. Frank Evans, Calhoun City, praised the membership "for the outstanding support of this profession-changing legislation."

The Mississippi State Medical Association brought a lawsuit related to the TPA legislation against the State of Mississippi and the Mississippi Board of

Optometry. The court dismissed the lawsuit with prejudice. The Association's legislative committee remained active, and focused its efforts on legislation for consumer protection, requiring insurers to include any willing provider in their health care plan.

During the 1990s there were several noteworthy accomplishments of MOA members. Dr. Ann Williams, Hattiesburg, served as president of the Association becoming the first woman to be elected to lead Mississippi Optometric Association. Dr. Lowell Jones, Indianola, became the fourth Mississippian to be elected president of the Southern Council of Optometry. Dr. John White, Baldwyn, was elected to a third term to the state senate.

Dr. Linda Johnson, Jackson, was not only named the National Optometric Association's 1996 Optometrist of the Year, but she was elected president of NOA the following year. Dr. Johnson also served as a member and as chairwoman of the Southern College of Optometry Board of Trustees.

Dr. James Moye, Laurel, and Dr. Eric Muir, Cleveland, were honored during the 1997 SCO Commencement on the anniversary of their fiftieth graduation. Both men were veterans of World War II and had faithfully served their patients and the association for over fifty years.

In 1997, a new Mission Statement was adopted committing the Association to:
1. improve visual healthcare and related systemic conditions
2. enhance optometric care through education
3. promote ethical standards
4. advance the profession of optometry
5. serve as an advocate for its members and the profession.

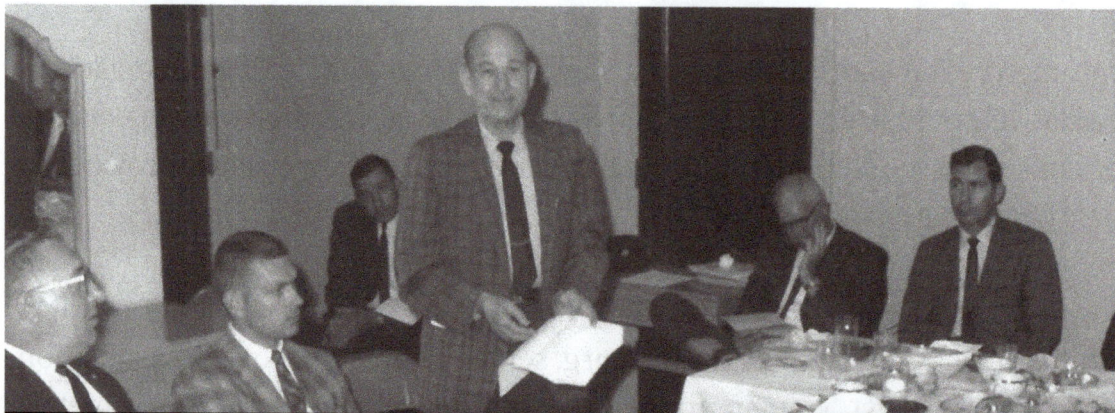
Richard Billups, MOA Attorney, giving legal and legislative update at MOA meeting.

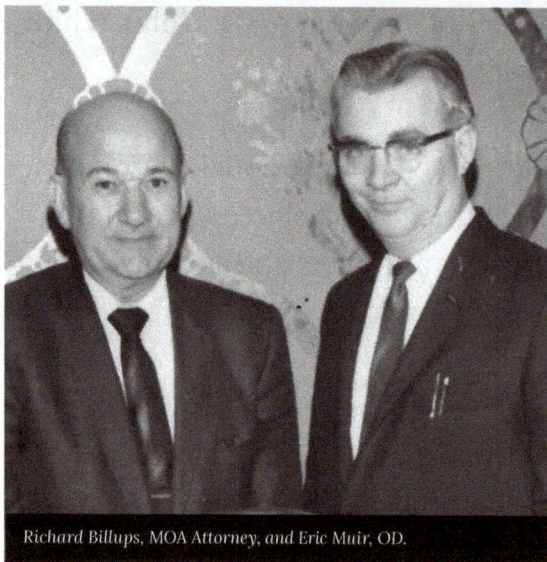
Richard Billups, MOA Attorney, and Eric Muir, OD.

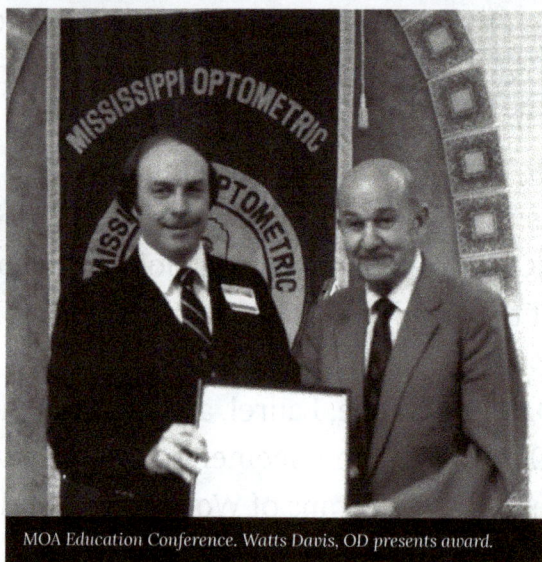
MOA Education Conference. Watts Davis, OD presents award.

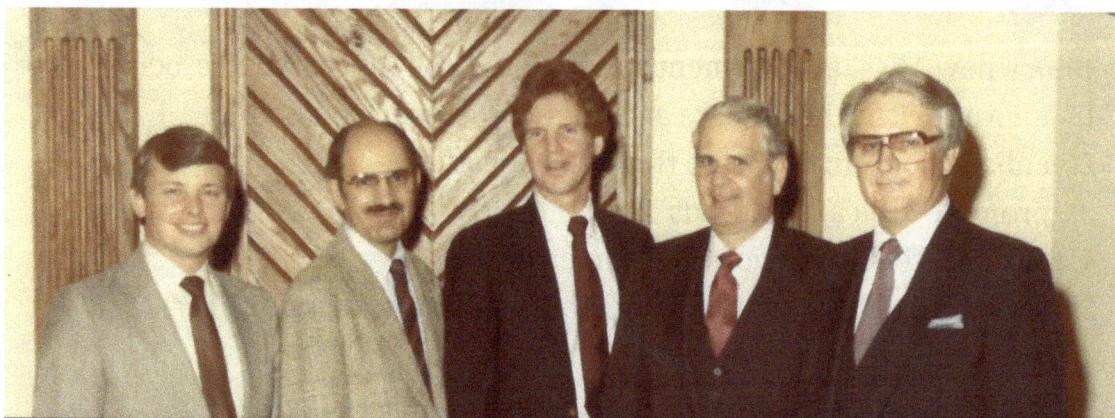
L-R: Earl Malone OD, Joe Joseph Od, James Brownlee OD, Gene Felder OD, George Martindale OD.

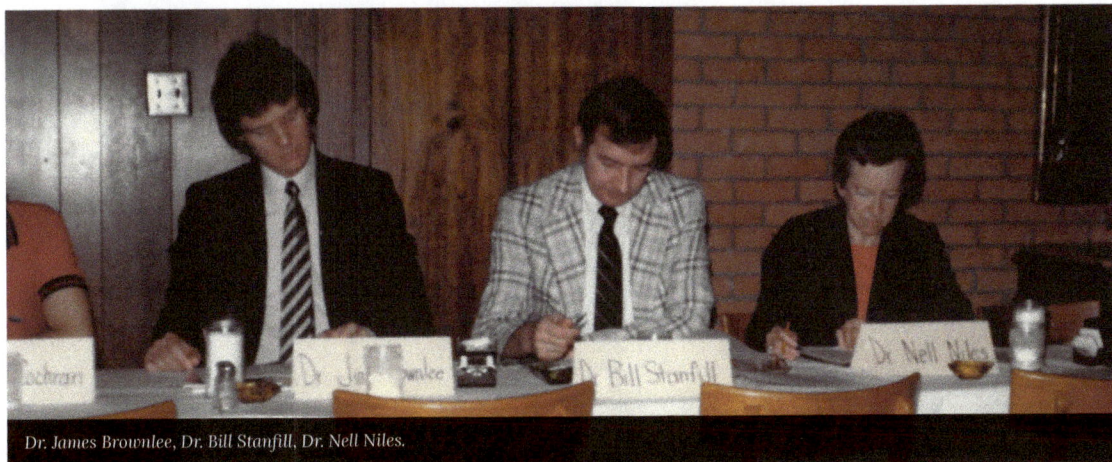

Dr. James Brownlee, Dr. Bill Stanfill, Dr. Nell Niles.

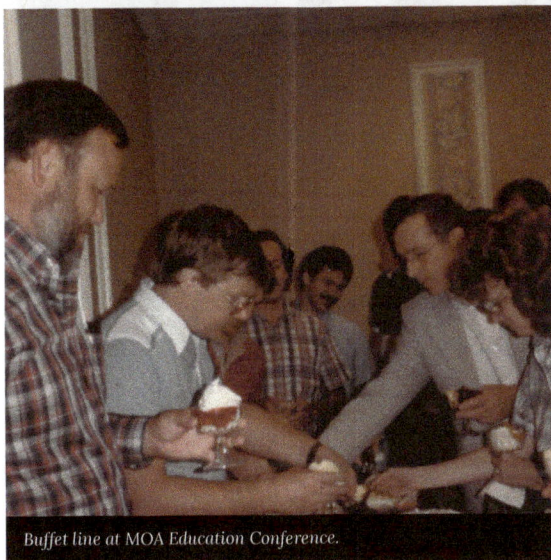

Buffet line at MOA Education Conference.

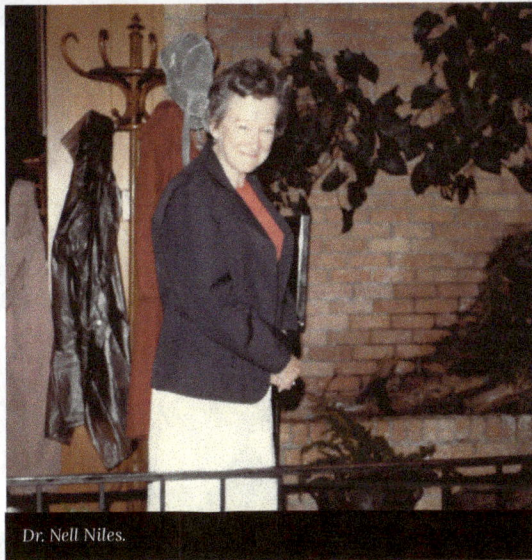

Dr. Nell Niles.

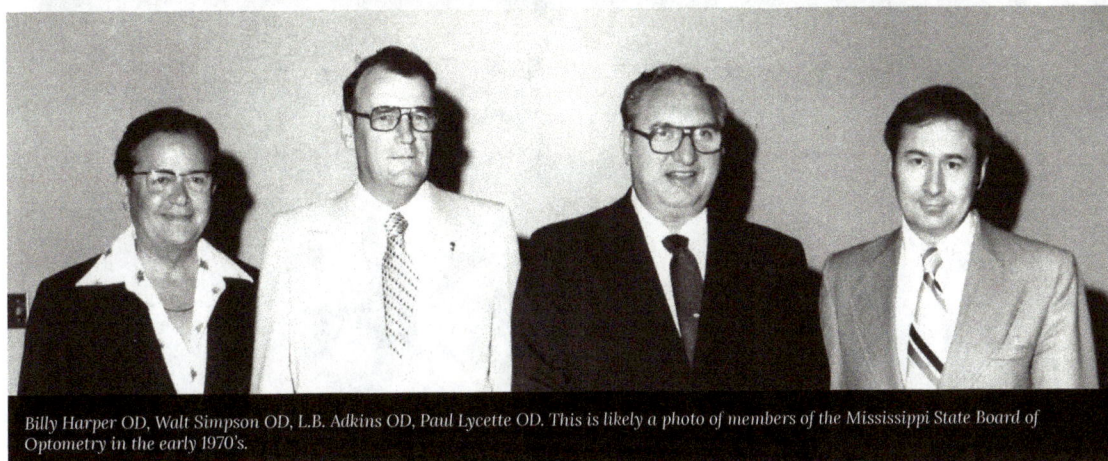

Billy Harper OD, Walt Simpson OD, L.B. Adkins OD, Paul Lycette OD. This is likely a photo of members of the Mississippi State Board of Optometry in the early 1970's.

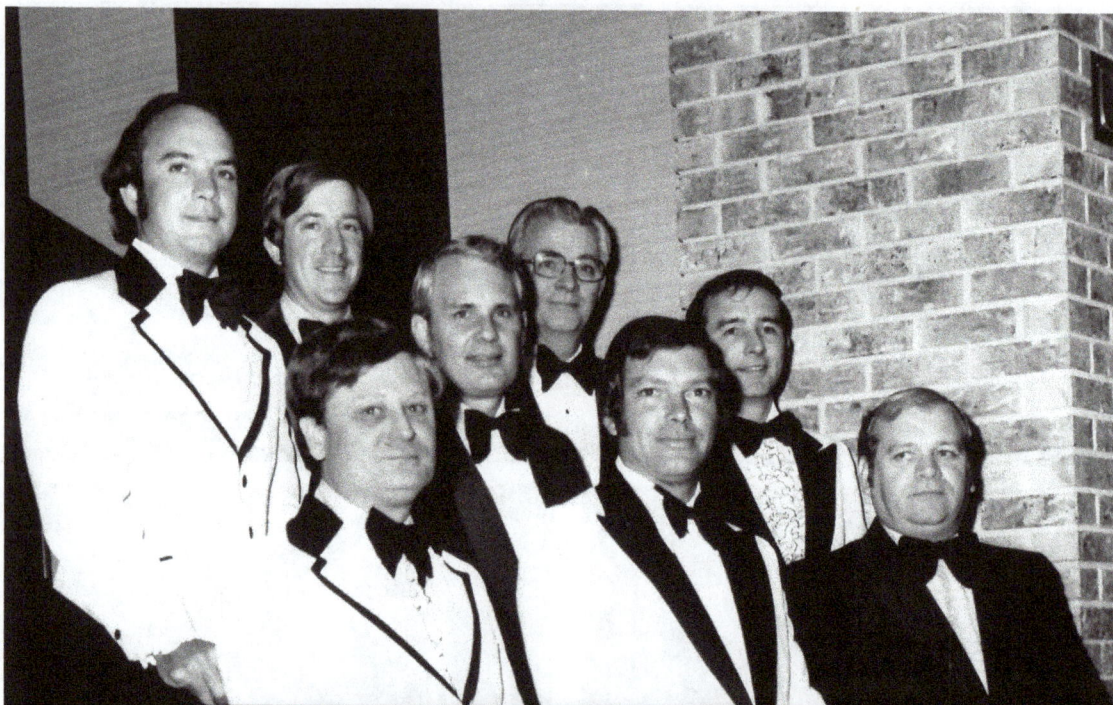

MOA Officers being installed in the mid-1970's. Front L-R: John White OD, Charlie Collins OD, Jim Herrington OD. Back L-R: Jerry Hollis OD, Billy Cochran OD, Gene Felder OD, Eric Muir OD, Bill Stanfill OD.

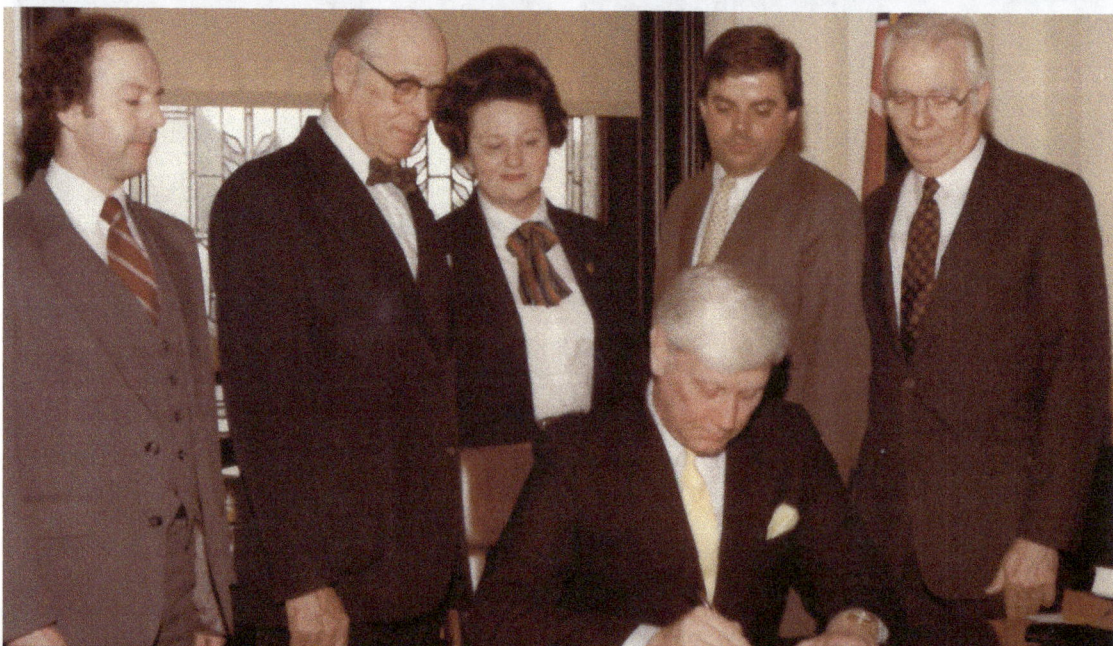

Governor William Allain signs the first permanent diagnostic pharmaceutical law in 1984. L-R: Larry Routt, OD; Avery McKinley, OD; Helen St. Clair. CAE; Clifford C. Thompson, attorney/lobbyist; Eric Muir, OD.

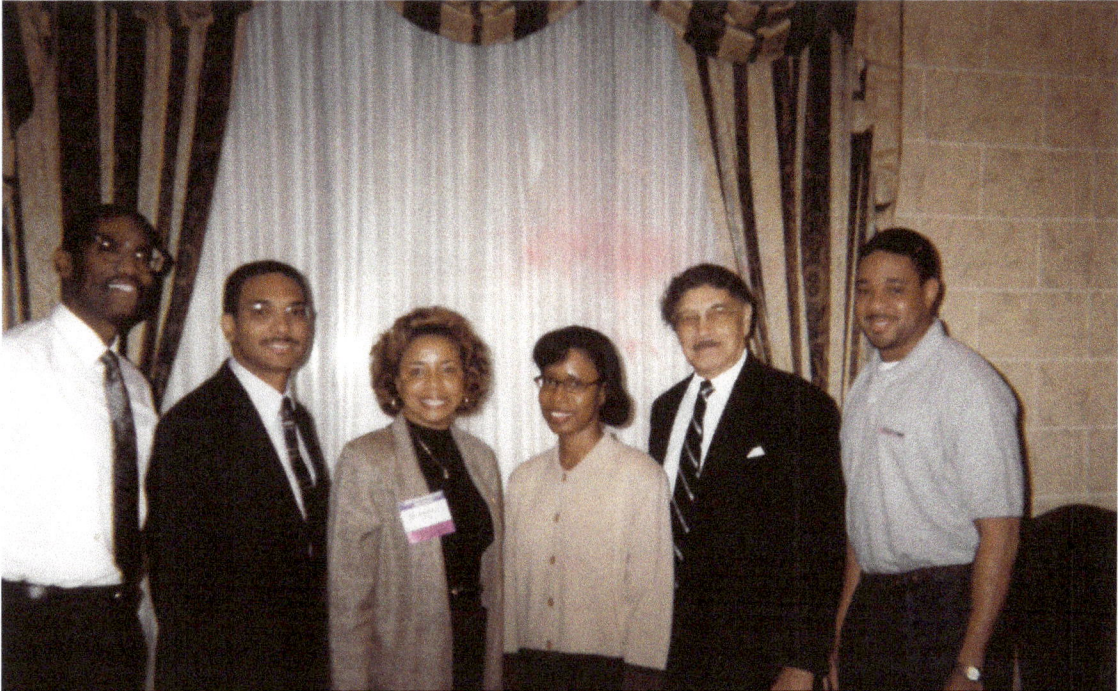

Mississippi Chapter of the National Optometric Association in the 1990's. L-R: Robert Lee OD, Dewey Handy OD, Linda Johnson OD, Jacquelyn Lucas OD, David W. White OD, Arthur "Reggie" Dampier OD.

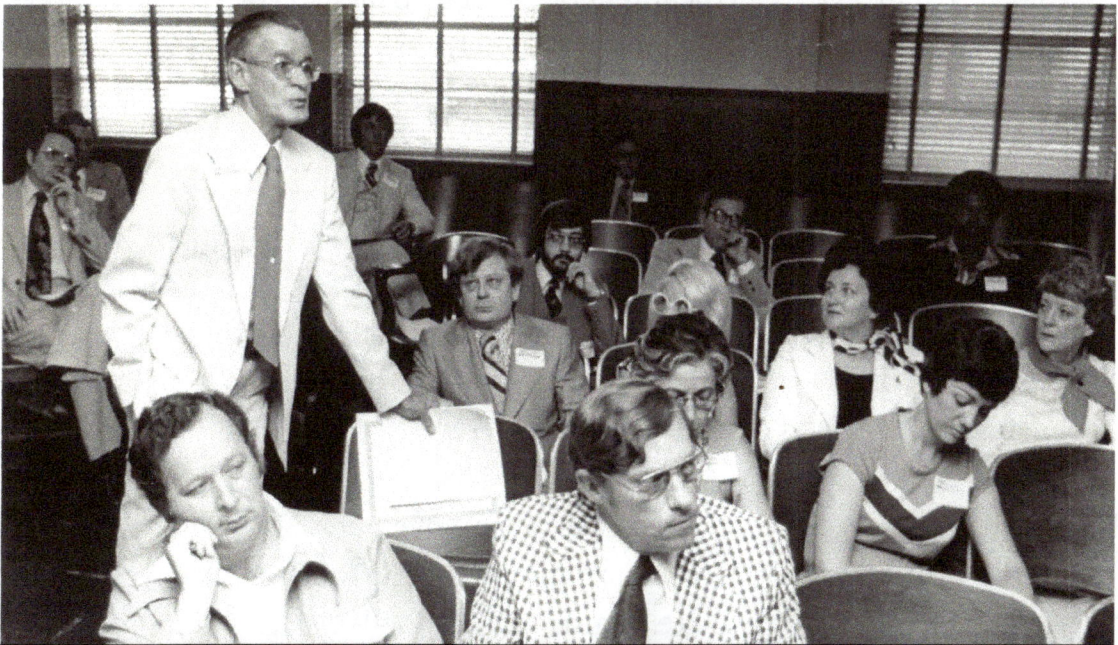

L-R. Standing, Senator Nap Cassibry. Immediately to Cassibry's right is Senator John White, OD. Two seats to the right of White is Helen St. Clair.

2000s

This decade began with one hundred and forty-three optometrists belonging to the Mississippi Optometric Association. The optical industry sponsors of the 2001 convention included: Alcon, Bayou Ophthalmic Instruments, Biocompatible Eyecare, Ciba, Focal Point, Future Optics, Helioasis, I Care Optical, Jackson Eye Institute, Kenmark, Mid-Gulf Instruments, Optical Distributors, Southern Optical, Topcom, and Tura. These are just a few of the many ophthalmic companies that have consistently supported the Association.

Legislation to update the Mississippi optometry law to the level of the surrounding states of Alabama, Arkansas, Louisiana, and Tennessee was introduced in 2002. The bill failed in the House Public Health & Welfare Committee. The state medical association sent a mailing to all of its members urging them to, "call today (to) tell your senator to protect patients from 'doctors' who didn't go to medical school. Don't give medical privileges to non-physicians. Kill any bill that would let optometrists prescribe schedule III, IV, or V drugs or perform surgery!"

Despite such opposition, Governor Haley Barbour signed SB 2682 on March 16, 2005, which authorized the use of oral pharmaceutical agents by licensed Mississippi optometrists. Association members did not quit either. Soon thereafter, the legislative committee recommended that the Association pursue the use of all oral medications, the ability to order lab tests, and the dispensing of medicated contact lenses.

The death of Dr. James P. Brownlee, Laurel, on November 22, 2004, was a great loss to the profession, and to Mississippi optometry. Dr. Brownlee was a past president, a member of the State Board, chair of the legislative committee for over ten years, and served as chair of various committees of the AOA. A year later, the Association's beloved Helen St. Clair suffered a stroke, and Linda Ross Aldy was appointed the third executive director of the Mississippi Optometric Association.

Many Association members were honored during the decade. Dr. Amy A. Crigler, Starkville, was named Mississippi's 2005 Optometrist of the Year, and Dr. Dewey Handy, Jackson, was named NOA's Optometrist of the Year. In 2004, the Association's long-serving assistant executive director, Barbara Smith, retired. In 2009, Dr. Linda Johnson, Jackson, was named the American Optometric Association's Optometrist of the Year, and Beverly Roberts was recognized as Paraoptometric of the Year. Dr. Larry Routt, Kosciusko, was recognized for his seven years of service as MOA's representative on the Medicaid Advisory Committee. Linda Ross Aldy earned her CAE certification.

The Association received a grant to participate in a pilot project called InfantSee. Later the program was adopted nationally and Governor Phil Bryant proclaimed the week of September 25 as InfantSee Week in Mississippi.

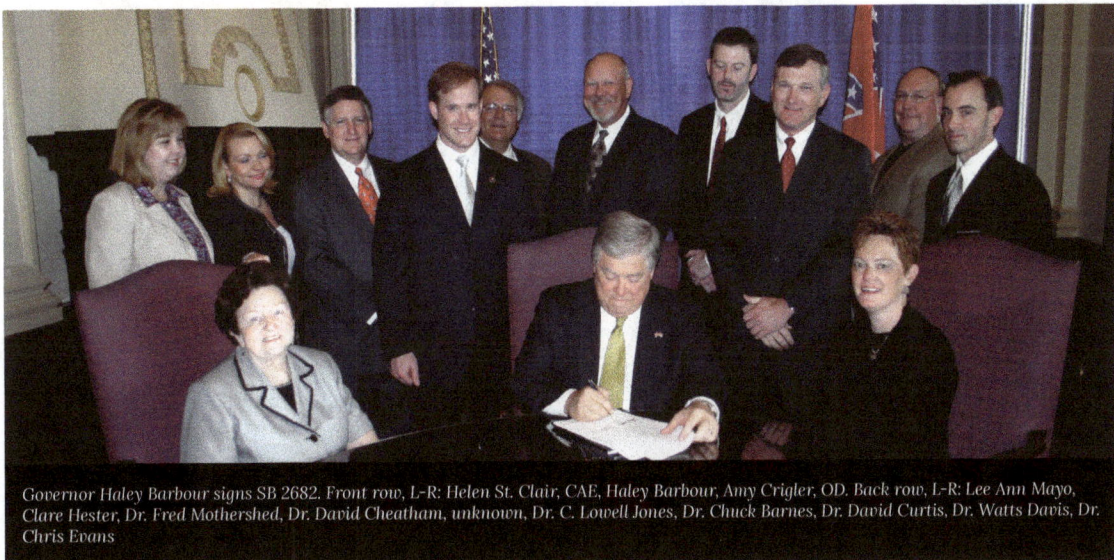

Governor Haley Barbour signs SB 2682. Front row, L-R: Helen St. Clair, CAE, Haley Barbour, Amy Crigler, OD. Back row, L-R: Lee Ann Mayo, Clare Hester, Dr. Fred Mothershed, Dr. David Cheatham, unknown, Dr. C. Lowell Jones, Dr. Chuck Barnes, Dr. David Curtis, Dr. Watts Davis, Dr. Chris Evans

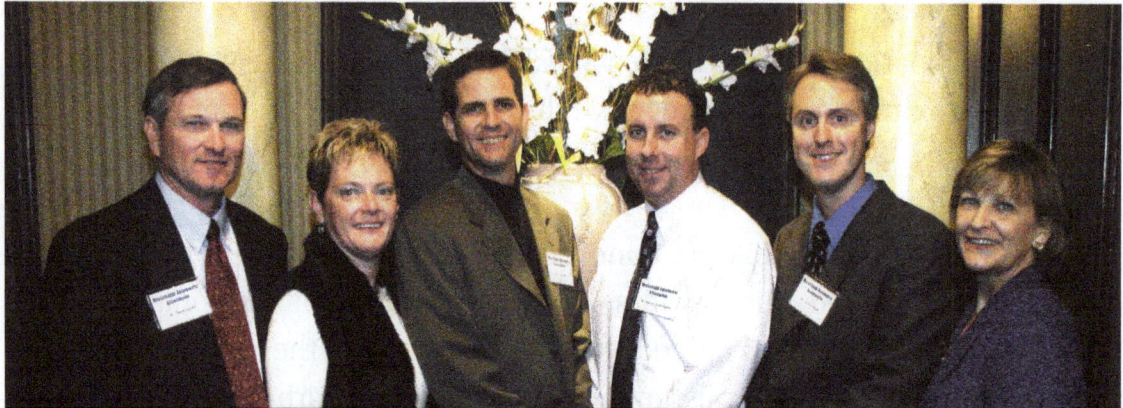

2006 Legislative Reception. L-R: David Curtis OD, Amy Crigler OD, Craig Belk OD, David Parker OD, Steven Reed OD, Linda Ross Aldy.

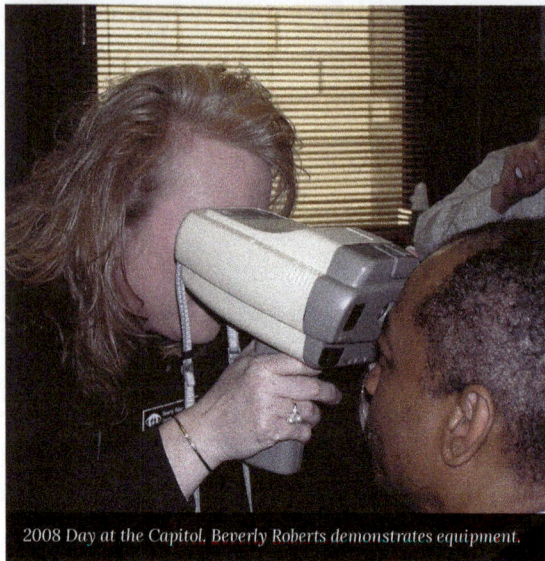

2008 Day at the Capitol. Beverly Roberts demonstrates equipment.

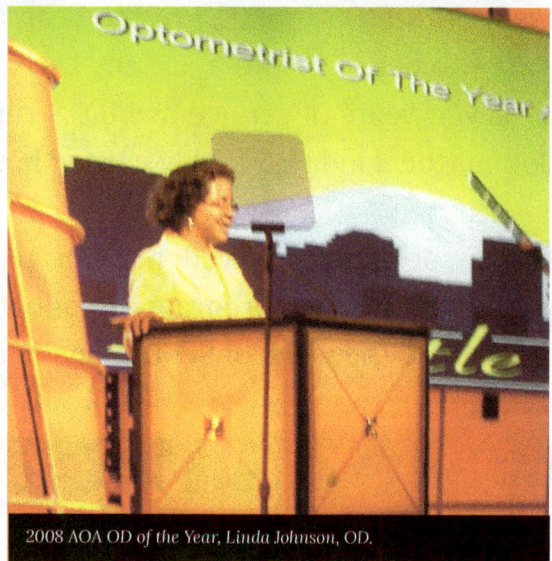

2008 AOA OD of the Year, Linda Johnson, OD.

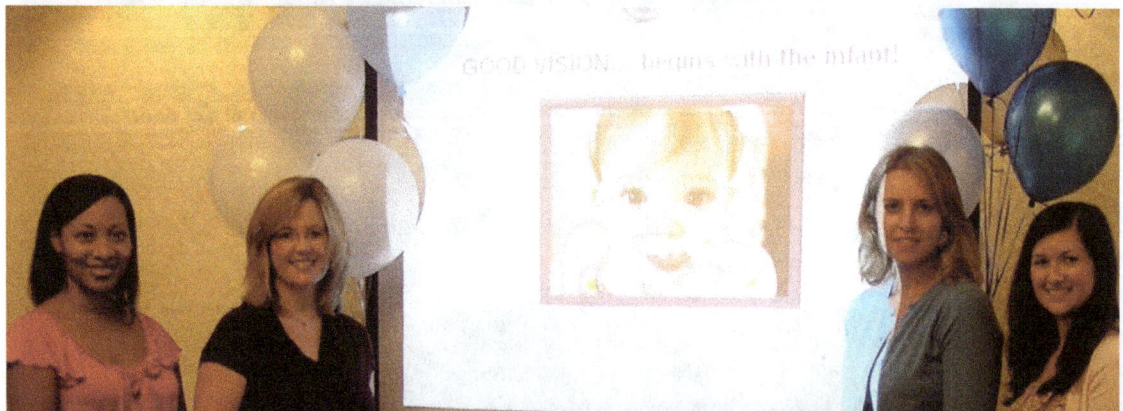

2005/2006, InfantSee Launch in Mississippi.

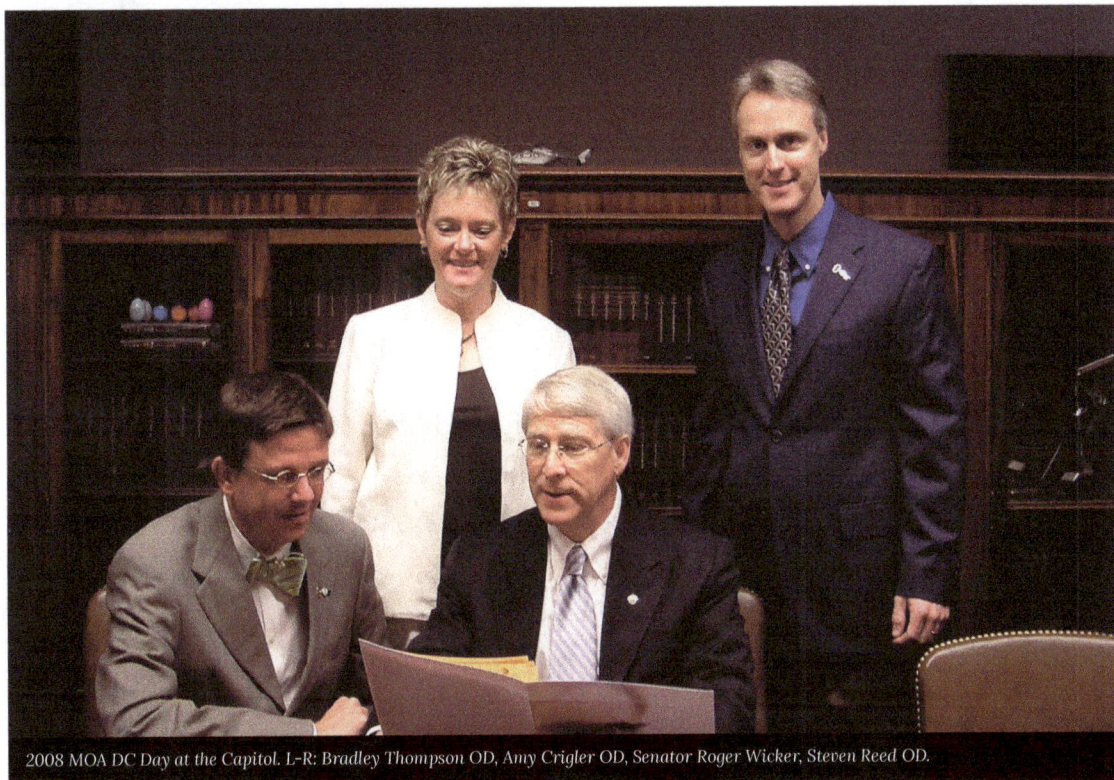

2008 MOA DC Day at the Capitol. L-R: Bradley Thompson OD, Amy Crigler OD, Senator Roger Wicker, Steven Reed OD.

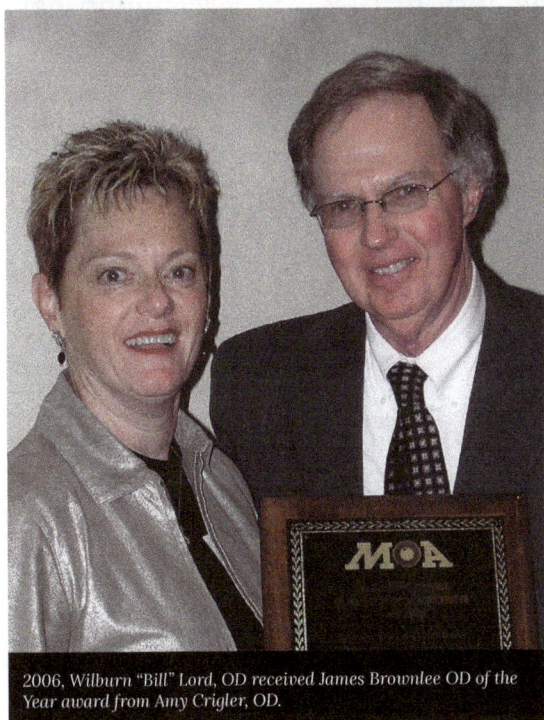

2006, Wilburn "Bill" Lord, OD received James Brownlee OD of the Year award from Amy Crigler, OD.

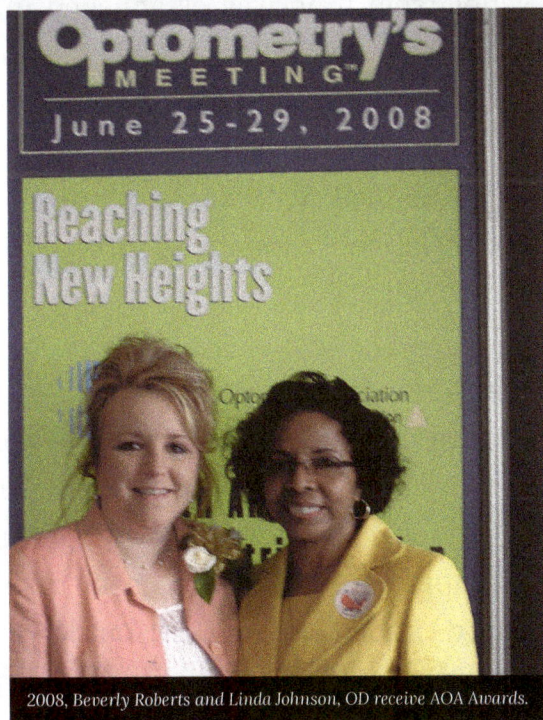

2008, Beverly Roberts and Linda Johnson, OD receive AOA Awards.

2010s

The decade leading up to the one hundred-year anniversary celebration of optometry in Mississippi revealed a growing and mature association expanding and accomplishing its Mission, which is: "to enhance, protect and promote the profession of optometry in Mississippi through advocacy, education, and advancing technology for patient eye care."

To accomplish the mission, the Association identified four main areas of concentration: communication, administration, advocacy, and membership. In 2015 the MOA and MVF partnered to offer no-cost eye exams to third graders who failed the new annual reading assessment. The kickoff event was held at the Mississippi Children's Museum in Jackson, and headlined by Lt. Governor Tate Reeves. In 2017, the Optometry for Progress PAC raised the most contributions in PAC history, $250,000.

A scholarship fund was established in memory of Helen St. Clair upon her passing October 31, 2013. The first scholarship was awarded in 2017.
Throughout the decade, many individuals were recognized for their contributions and accomplishments. Sarah E. Link, associate executive director, earned her CAE certification. Dr. Steven Reed, Magee, became the first Mississippi optometrist to be elected to the AOA Board of Trustees. Dr. David Parker, Olive Branch, was elected to the Mississippi Senate.

Linda Ross Aldy, executive director, was installed as president of the International Association of Optometric Executives, or IAOE. The association commended Dr. Mark Tomsik, Moss Point, and Dr. Larry Routt, Kosciusko, for articles published in optometric journals. For the second year in a row, the Mississippi Paraoptometric Association won all three national awards. And Leonard Farmer, Optical Distributors, was recognized for forty years of service and support of the Association and the profession of optometry.

The Association continued to help pass legislation in keeping with its mission. The medicated contact lens bill became law July 1, 2010. In 2019, the Children's Vision bill, HB 1322, was signed into law by Governor Phil Bryant. The Association's legislative committee was restructured into three regions, with each having one to two key persons.

Since its establishment in 1960, The Mississippi Vision Foundation has engaged in and worked for the improvement of vision and eye care by establishing optometric research and educational programs, providing scholarships for those seeking to join the optometric profession, and by offering indigent eye care programs. Current projects include Third Grade Eye Exams; Vision USA, *InfantSEE*, and the Helen St. Clair Scholarship Fund.

In an effort to prepare future leaders of the Mississippi Optometric Association, the Leadership Optometry Program was initiated in 2015. To date there are approximately twenty-five graduates of the program, and all are in leadership positions in the Association. In 2018, the Association established marketing and branding campaigns designed to educate the general public, teachers, and legislators on the importance of regular eye and vision exams, and the need for a family optometrist. As part of the campaign, the Association's logo was redesigned and has been enthusiastically received by the membership. At the end of the decade, the total membership of the Mississippi Optometric Association, including students, stood at three hundred and twelve.

As the One Hundred Anniversary came to a close, MOA's Executive Director for the past fifteen years, Linda Ross Aldy, related that working with Mississippi optometry is like working with family. The highlight of her tenure has been the continued expansion of the scope of practice, and watching the growth of members of the Association in leadership roles at the local, state, and national level.

Dr. Amy A. Crigler, Starkville, commented as she was completing her second term as MOA president in 2019: "The Association is in a much better place than it was the last time (2007) I was president." Her remark sums up the one hundred years of Mississippi optometry history. The profession is in a much better place than it was in 1920.

Postscript

During the 2021 session of the Mississippi Legislature, HB 1302 was passed and signed into law by Governor Tate Reeves. Dr. Ryan Wally, MOA Legislative Chairman, summarized the bill: "HB 1302 includes oral steroids, pharmaceuticals to schedule 2-5, injectable authority, and other Primary Eyecare Procedures (PEP), including YAG laser posterior capsulotomy, and removal of presumed non-cancerous lesions."

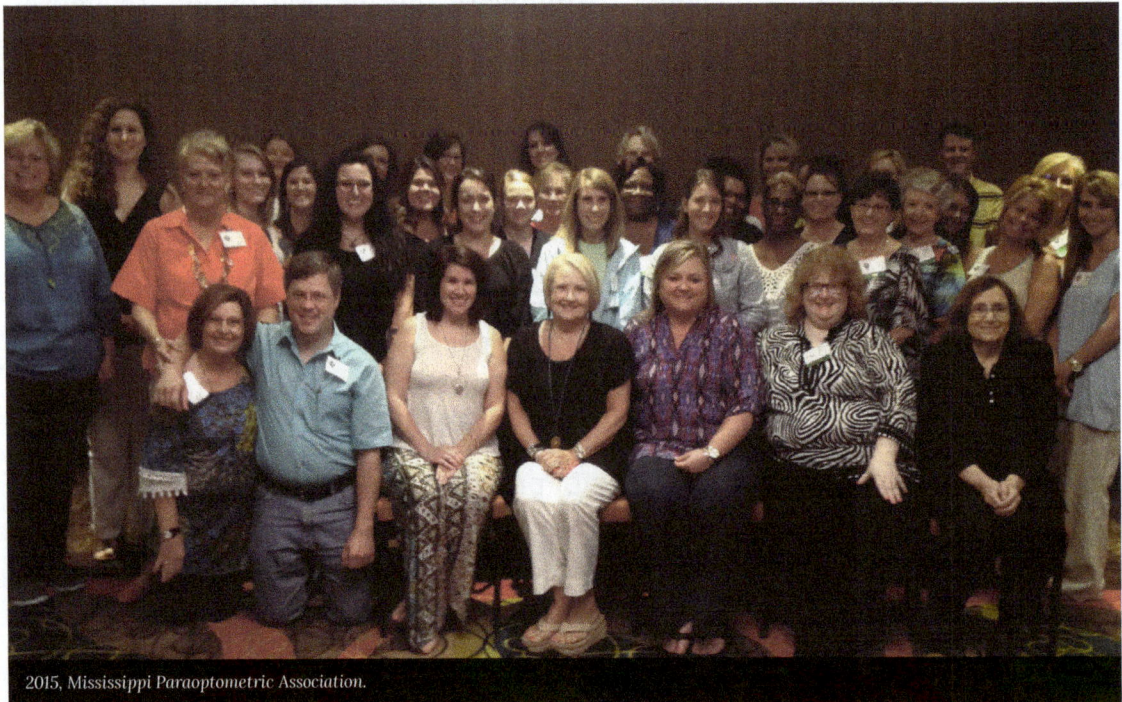

2015, Mississippi Paraoptometric Association.

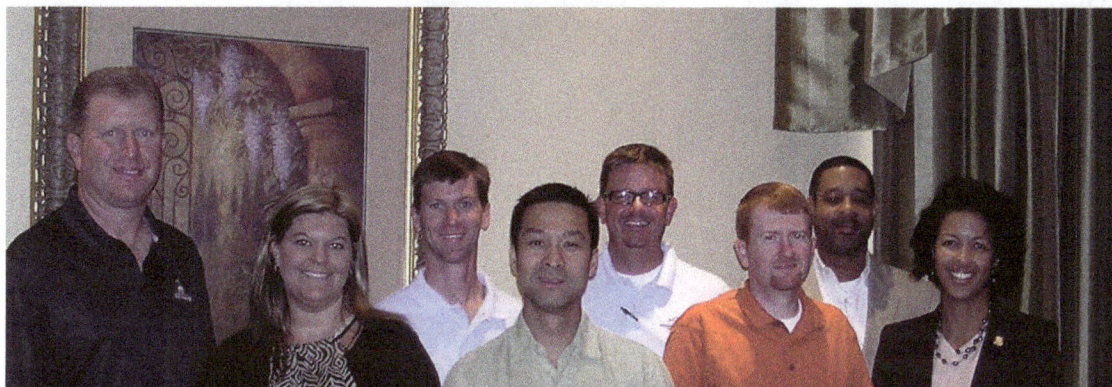

2011, MOA Board with AOA Trustee. L-R: Mike Weeden OD, Allison Lord OD, Philip Marler OD, Minh Duong OD, Bradley Thompson OD, Eric Randle OD, Arthur "Reggie" Dampier OD, Hillary Hawthorne OD.

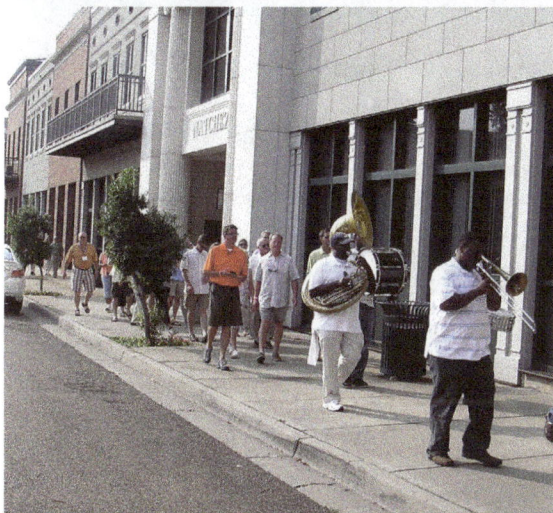

2011 Natchez Pub Crawl at Summer Convention.

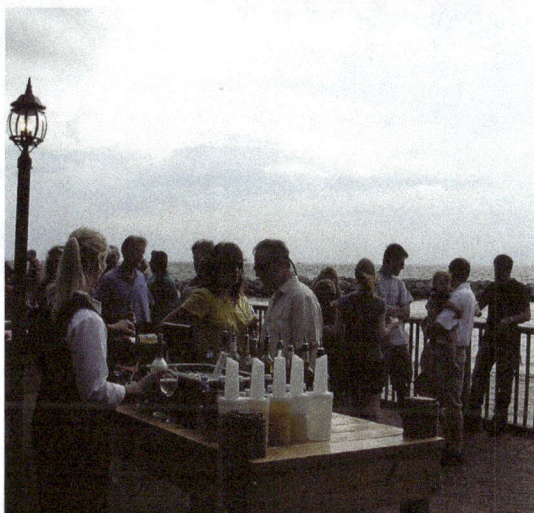

2012 Point Clear Reception at Summer Convention.

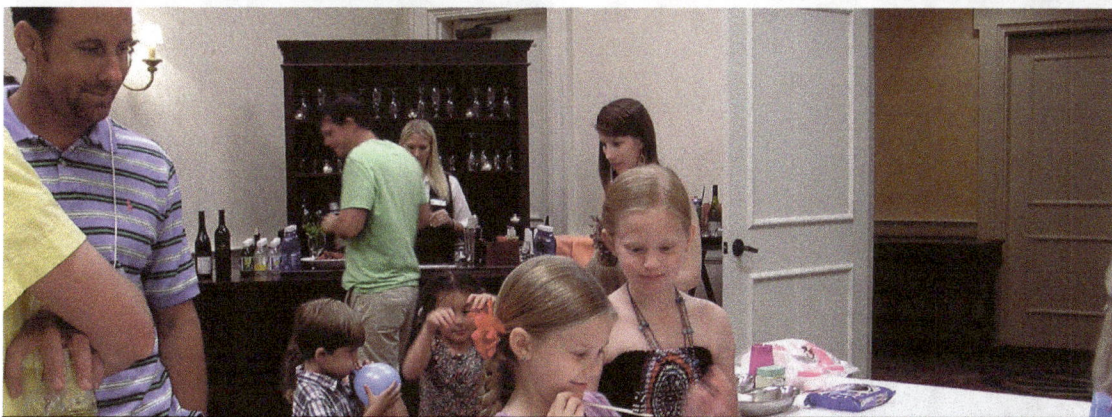

2012 Summer Convention in Point Clear, AL..

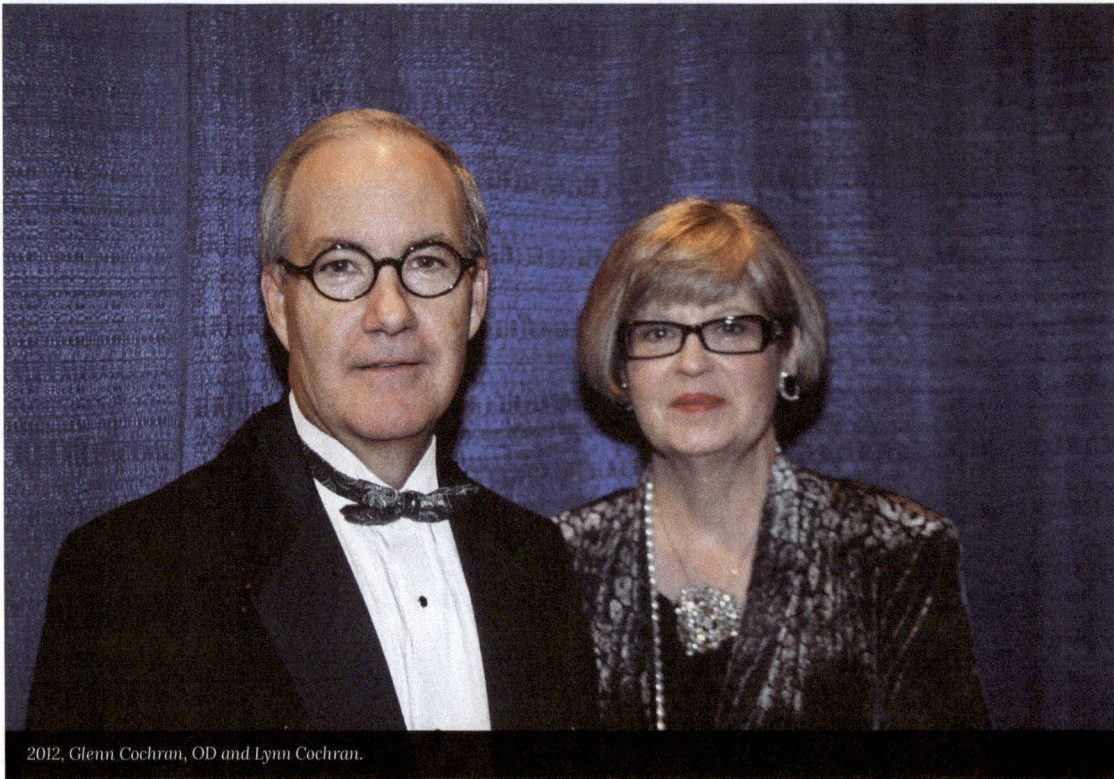

2012, Glenn Cochran, OD and Lynn Cochran.

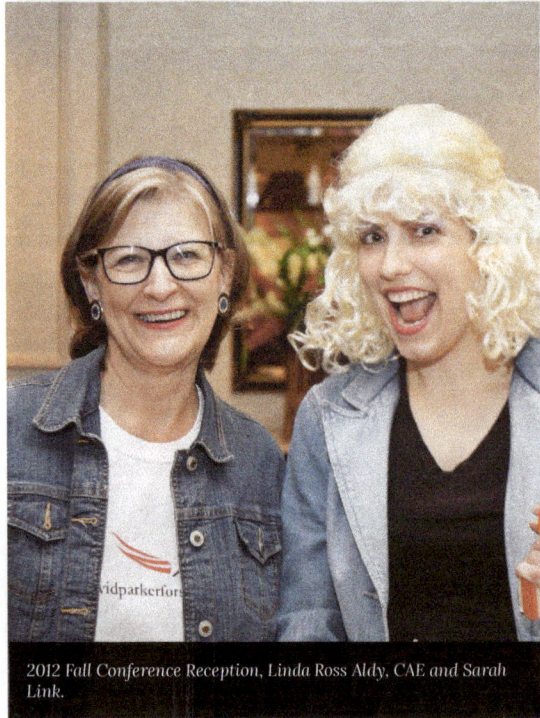

2012 Fall Conference Reception, Linda Ross Aldy, CAE and Sarah Link.

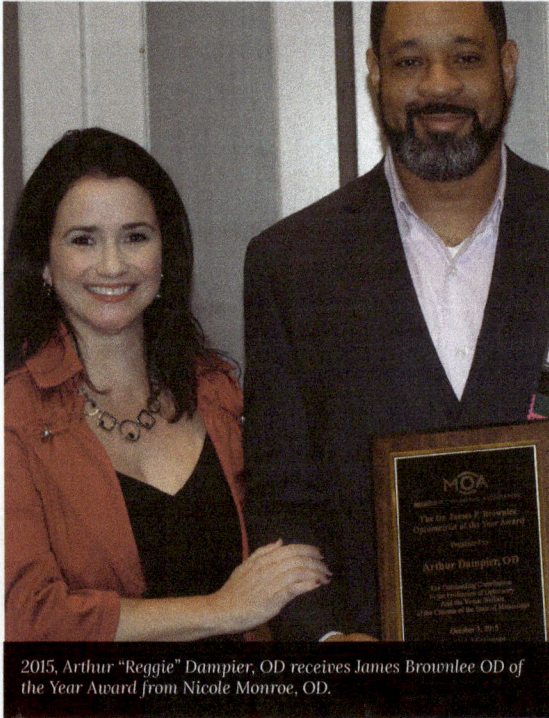

2015, Arthur "Reggie" Dampier, OD receives James Brownlee OD of the Year Award from Nicole Monroe, OD.

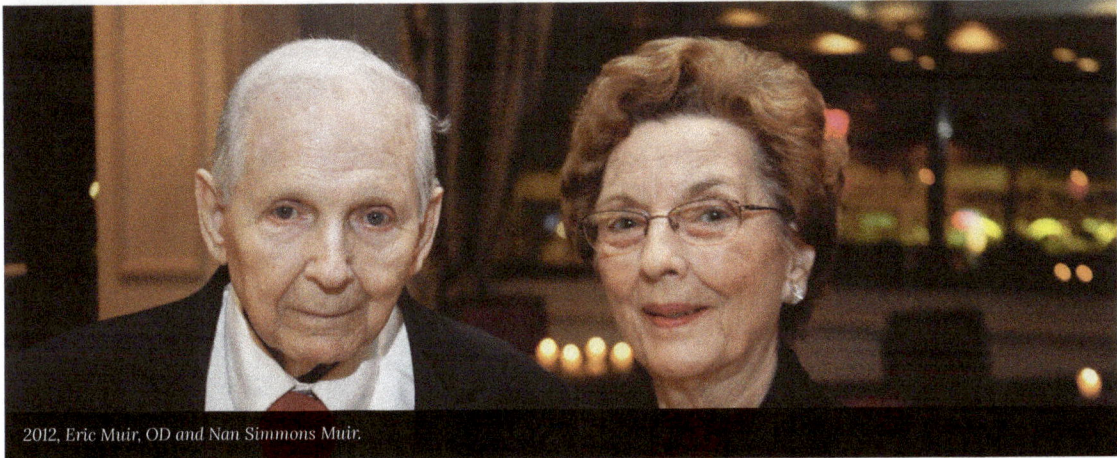

2012, Eric Muir, OD and Nan Simmons Muir.

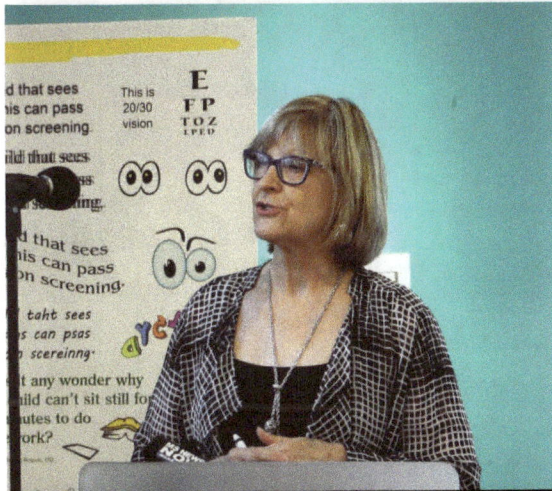

2015, Linda Ross Aldy, CAE at the Mississippi Children's Museum for the 3rd Grade Eye Exam Program launch.

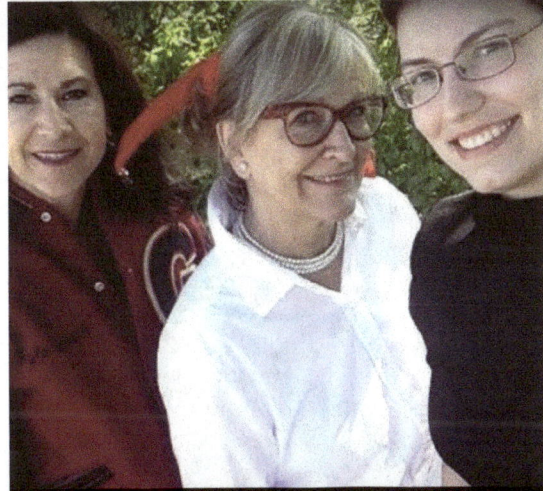

2015, Sheila Gonseth, Linda Ross Aldy, CAE and Sarah Link preparing for the Fall Conference Sock Hop reception.

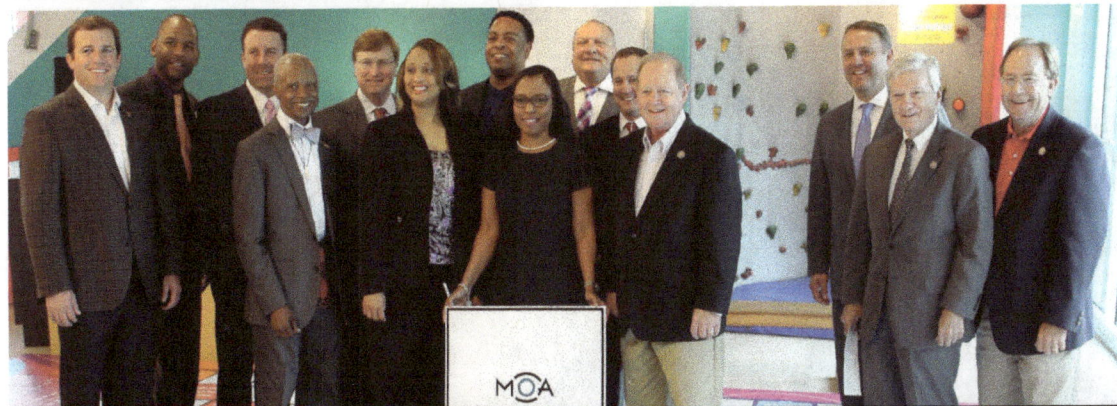

2015, Legislators and Optometrists at the Mississippi Children's Museum for the 3rd Grade Eye Exam Program launch.

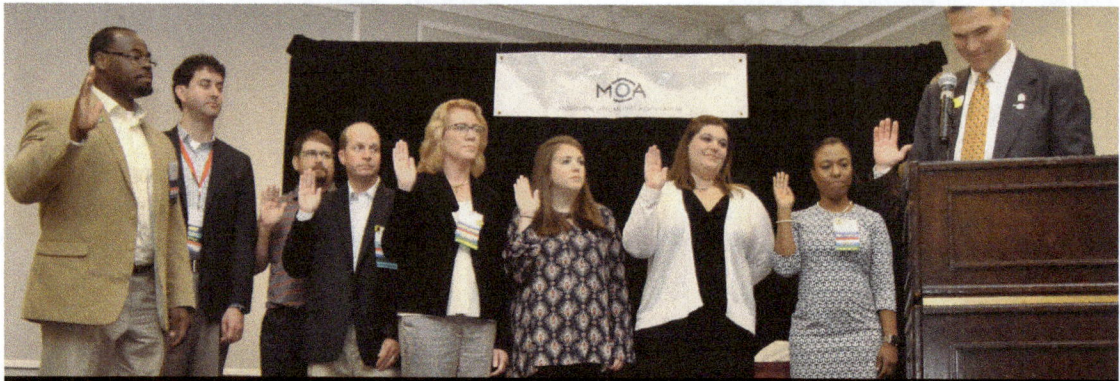

2015, MOA Board sworn in by AOA Trustee. L-R: Chris Bullin OD, Ryan Wally OD, Jason "Bo" Beddingfield OD, Evan Davis OD, Lori Blackmer OD, Mary Kathryn Wilson OD, Allison Lord OD, Tonyatta Hairston OD, Robert Layman OD.

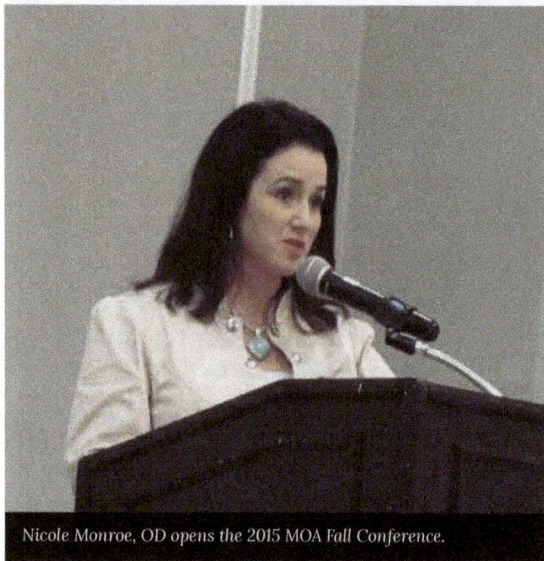

Nicole Monroe, OD opens the 2015 MOA Fall Conference.

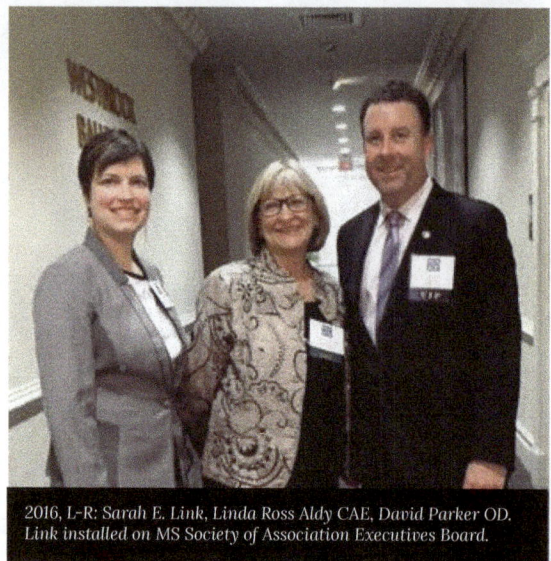

2016, L-R: Sarah E. Link, Linda Ross Aldy CAE, David Parker OD. Link installed on MS Society of Association Executives Board.

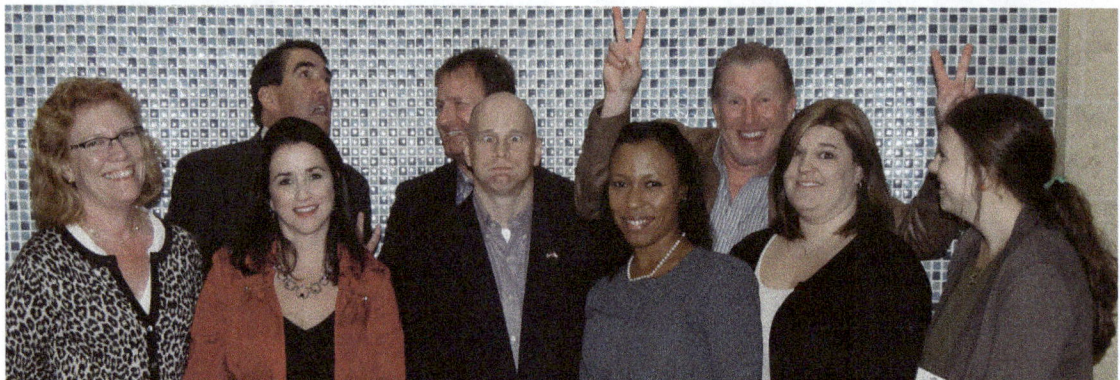

2016 MOA Board. L-R Front: Lori Blackmer OD, Nicole Monroe OD, Greg Loose OD, Tonyatta Hairston OD, Allison Lord OD, Mary Kathryn Wilson OD. L-R Back: Jim DeVleming OD (AOA Trustee), Dax Eckard OD, Mike Weeden OD.

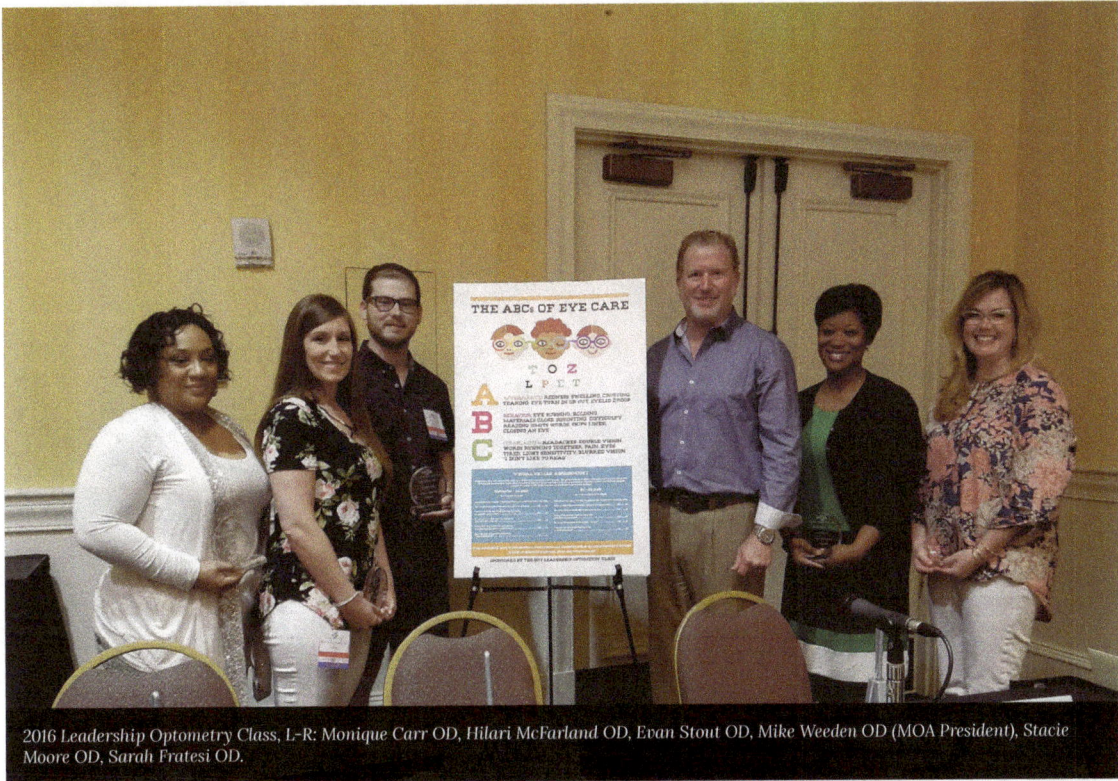

2016 Leadership Optometry Class, L-R: Monique Carr OD, Hilari McFarland OD, Evan Stout OD, Mike Weeden OD (MOA President), Stacie Moore OD, Sarah Fratesi OD.

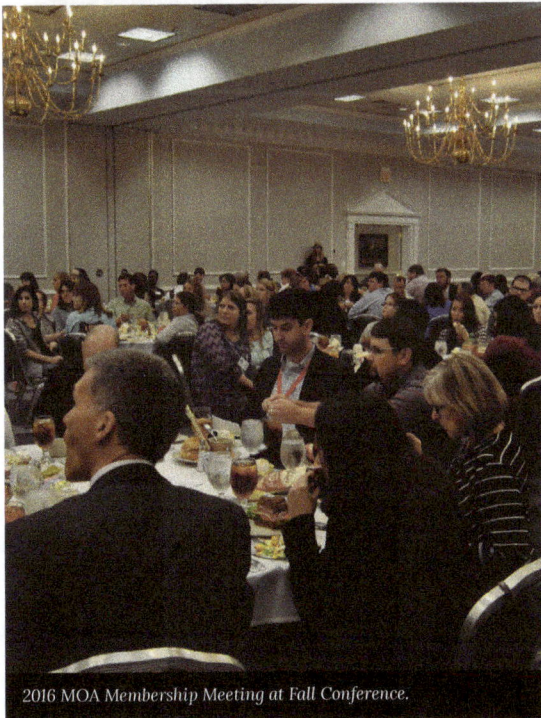

2016 MOA Membership Meeting at Fall Conference.

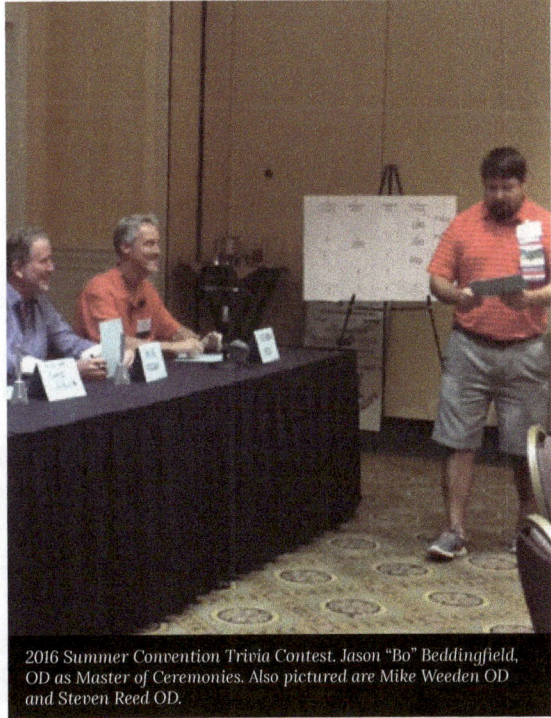

2016 Summer Convention Trivia Contest. Jason "Bo" Beddingfield, OD as Master of Ceremonies. Also pictured are Mike Weeden OD and Steven Reed OD.

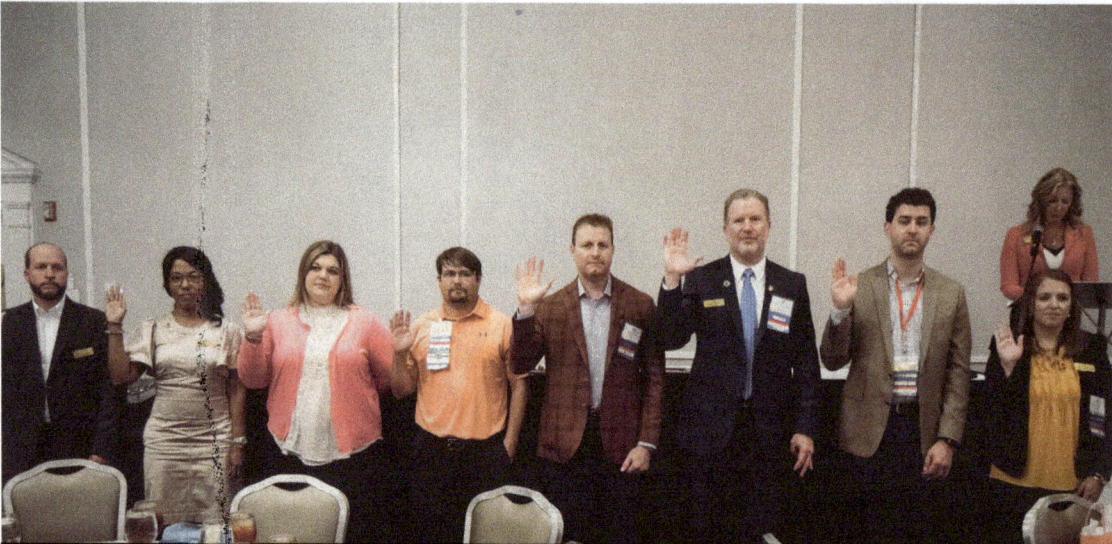

2017 MOA Board sworn in by AOA Trustee. L–R: Evan Davis OD, Tonyatta Hairston OD, Allison Lord Griffin OD, Jason "Bo" Beddingfield OD, Dax Eckard OD, Mike Weeden OD, Ryan Wally OD, Mary Kathryn Wilson OD, Barbara Horn, OD.

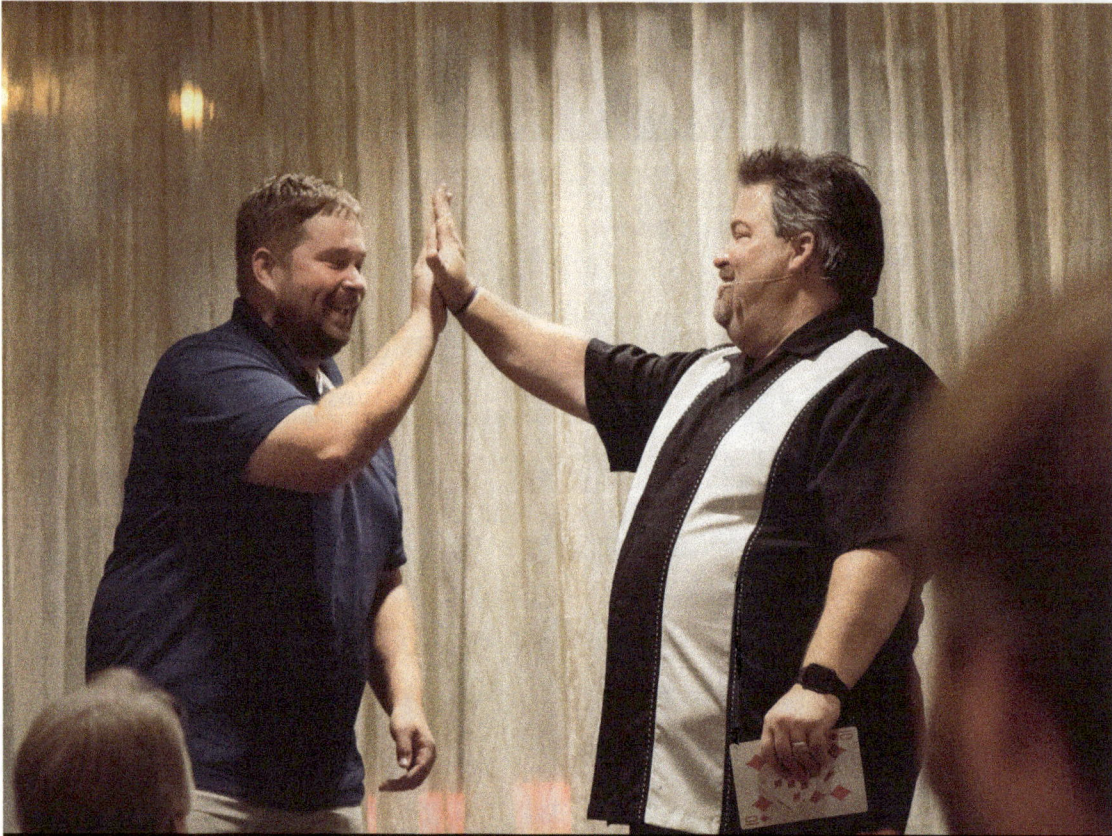

2017 Fall Conference Welcome Reception. L–R: Josh Bostick, OD with magician Dorian LaChance.

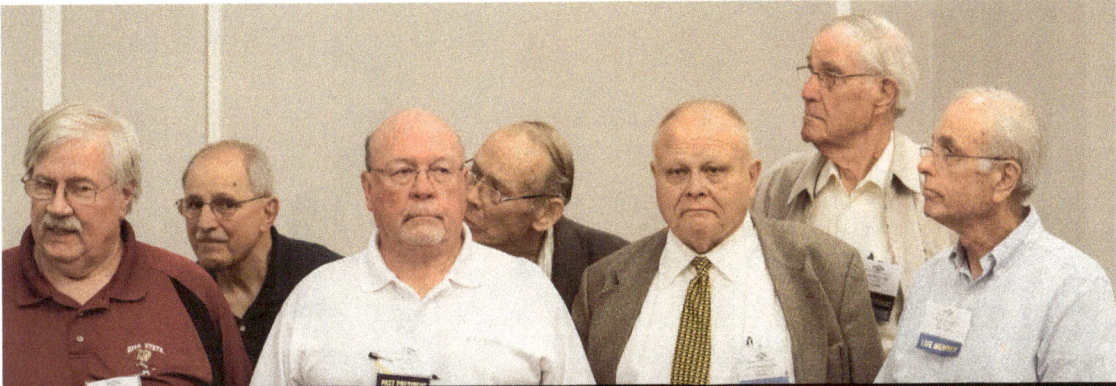

2017, MOA Life Members at Fall Conference. L-R: Frank Reese OD, Joe Joseph OD, Watts Davis OD, Bernard Ellis OD, W. C. Maples OD, John Mohr OD, John W. Turner OD.

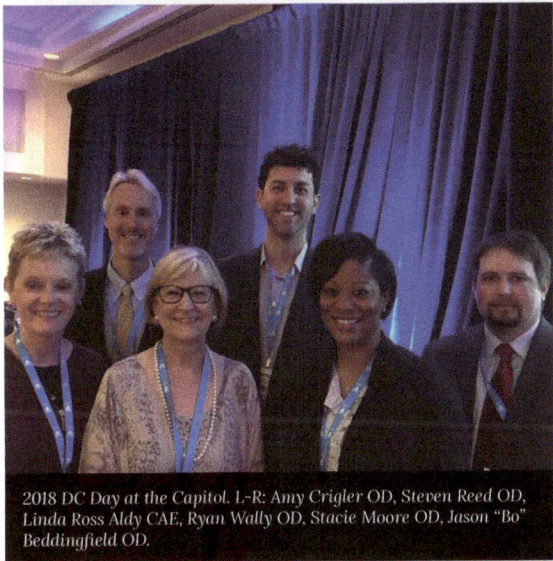

2018 DC Day at the Capitol. L-R: Amy Crigler OD, Steven Reed OD, Linda Ross Aldy CAE, Ryan Wally OD, Stacie Moore OD, Jason "Bo" Beddingfield OD.

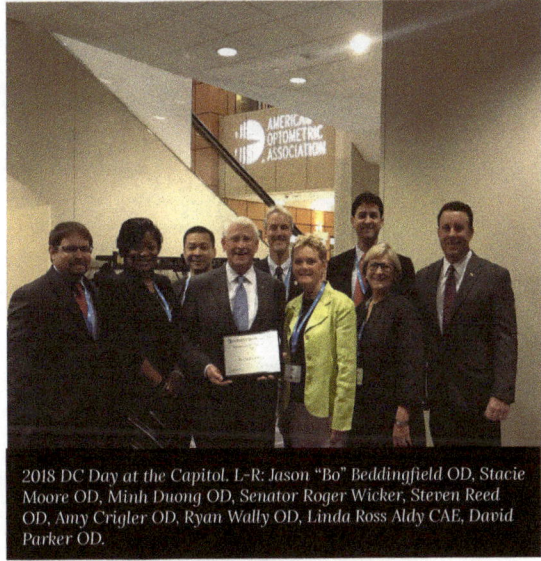

2018 DC Day at the Capitol. L-R: Jason "Bo" Beddingfield OD, Stacie Moore OD, Minh Duong OD, Senator Roger Wicker, Steven Reed OD, Amy Crigler OD, Ryan Wally OD, Linda Ross Aldy CAE, David Parker OD.

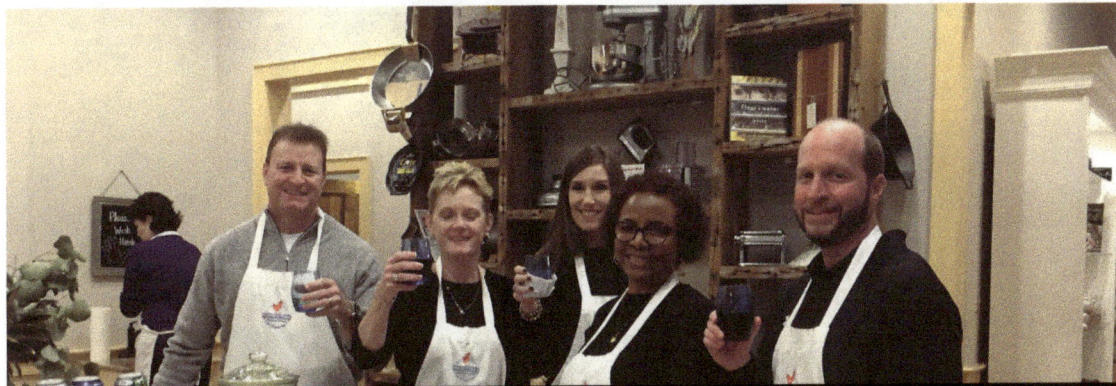

2018 MOA Board Retreat and Strategic Planning, at the Livingston Cooking School. L-R: Dax Eckard OD, Amy Crigler OD, Hilari McFarland OD, Linda Johnson OD, Evan Davis OD.

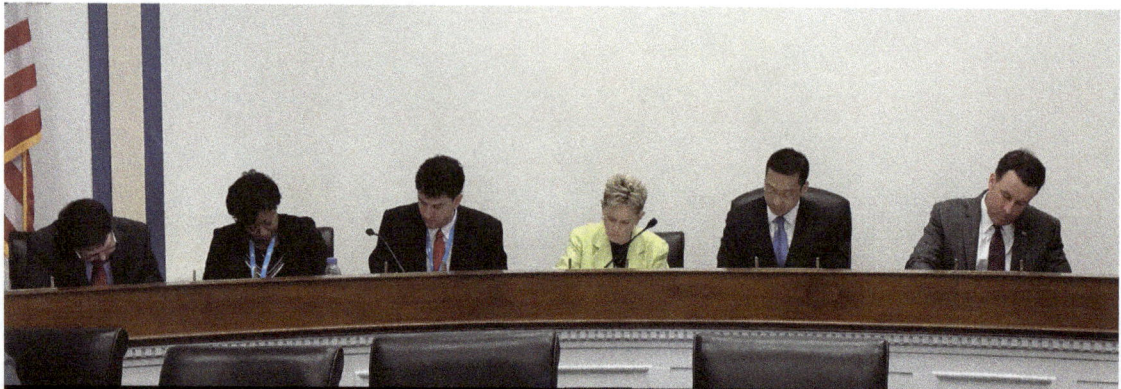

2018 DC Day at the Capitol, MOA representatives hard at work writing thank you notes to the congressional delegation. L-R: Jason "Bo" Beddingfield OD, Stacie Moore OD, Ryan Wally OD, Amy Crigler OD, Minh Duong OD, David Parker OD.

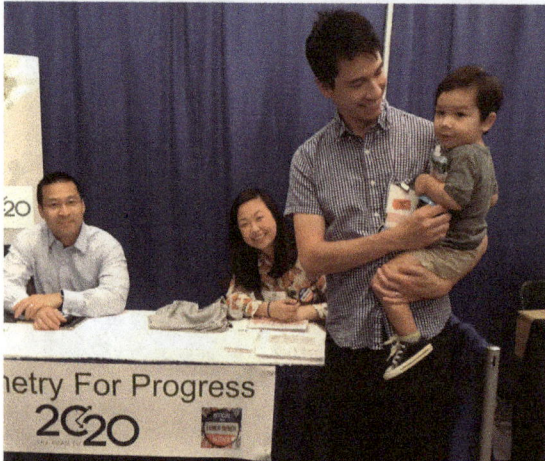

2018 Fall Conference, OFP PAC Booth. L-R: Minh Duong OD, PAC Chair. Tiffany McElroy OD, Grassroots Chair. Justin McElroy, OD with son Henry McElroy.

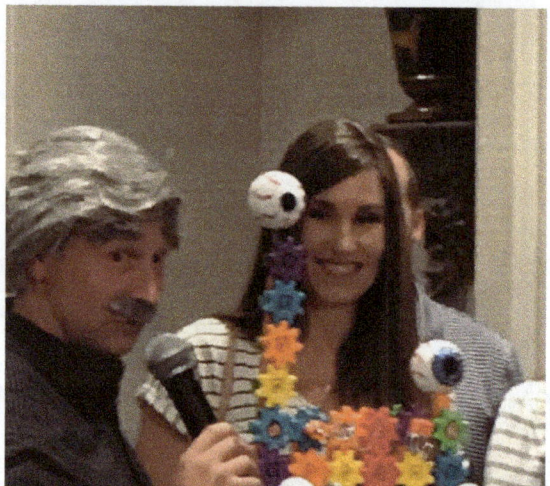

2018 Fall Conference Welcome Reception. L-R: Greg Loose OD, Hilari McFarland OD, Mandi Smith OD.

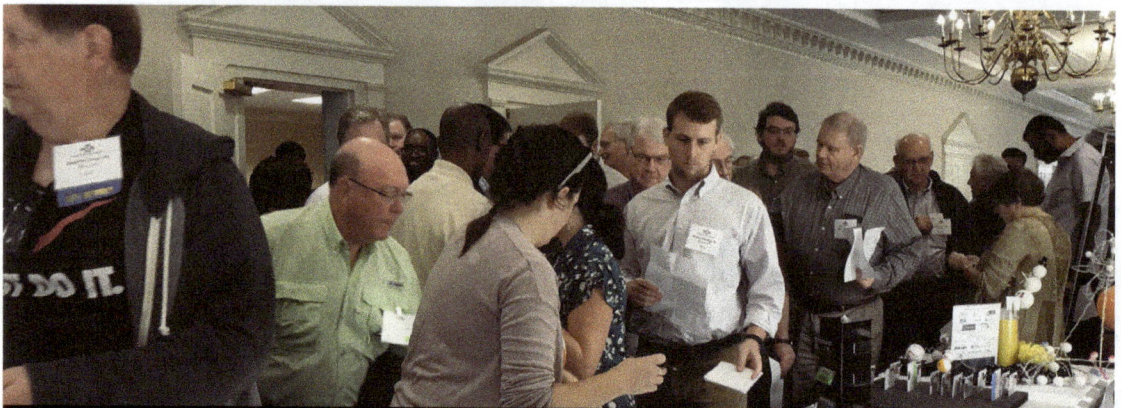

2018 Fall Conference Registration Desk, scanning and stamping CE papers.

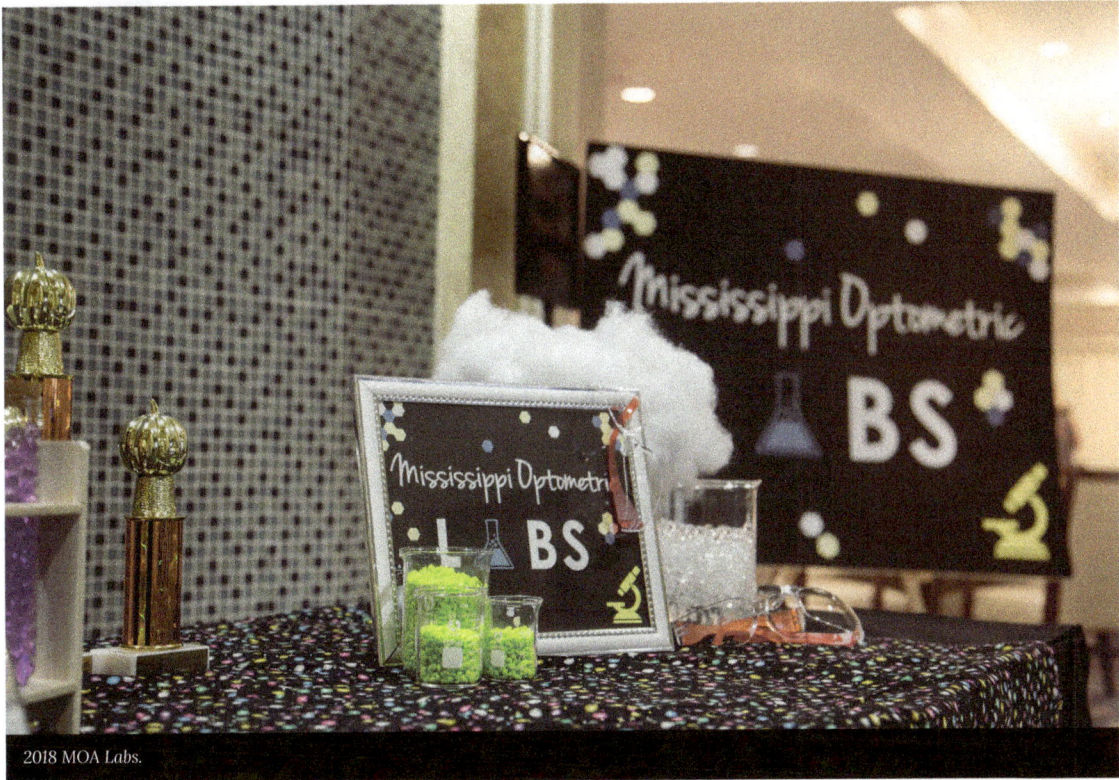

2018 MOA Labs.

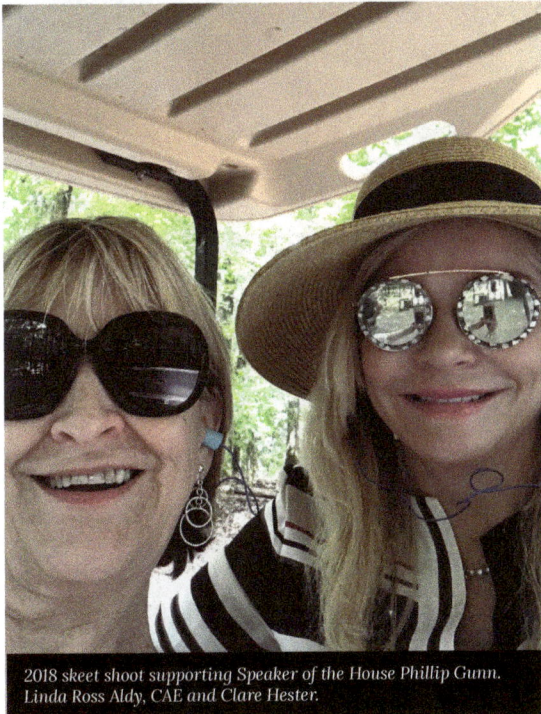

2018 skeet shoot supporting Speaker of the House Phillip Gunn.
Linda Ross Aldy, CAE and Clare Hester.

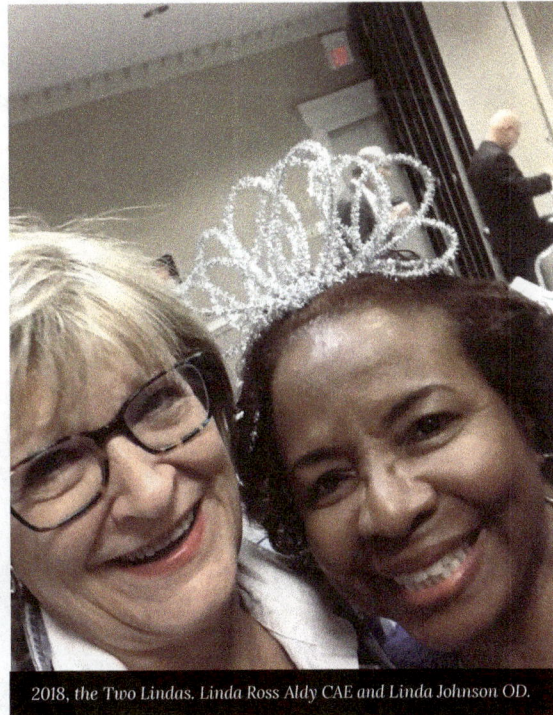

2018, the Two Lindas. Linda Ross Aldy CAE and Linda Johnson OD.

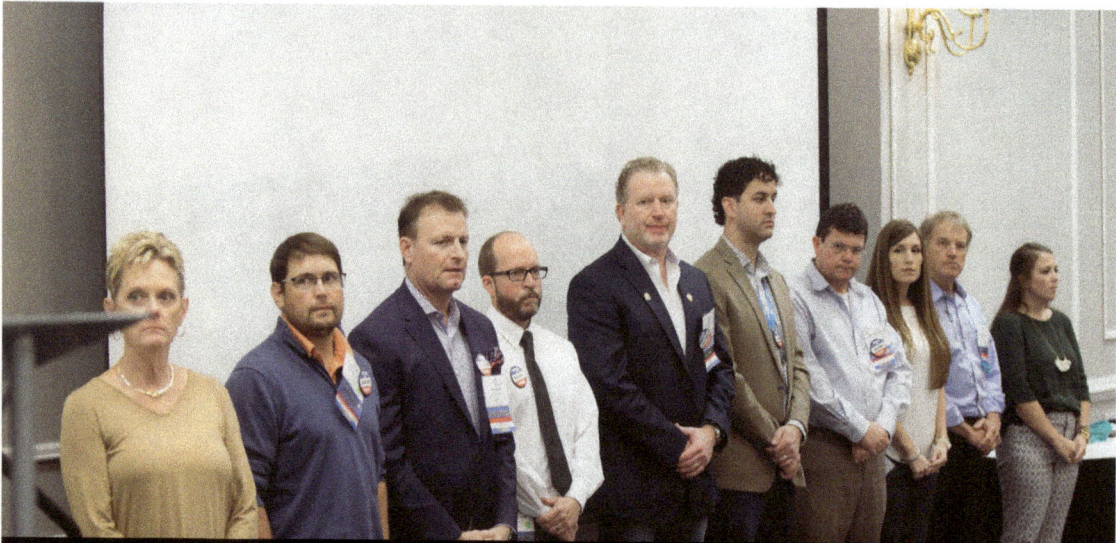

2018 MOA Board sworn in. L-R: Amy Crigler OD, Jason "Bo" Beddingfield OD, Dax Eckard OD, Evan Davis OD, Mike Weeden OD, Ryan Wally OD, Jacob Irey OD, Hilari McFarland OD, Rod Fields OD, Mary Kathryn Wilson OD.

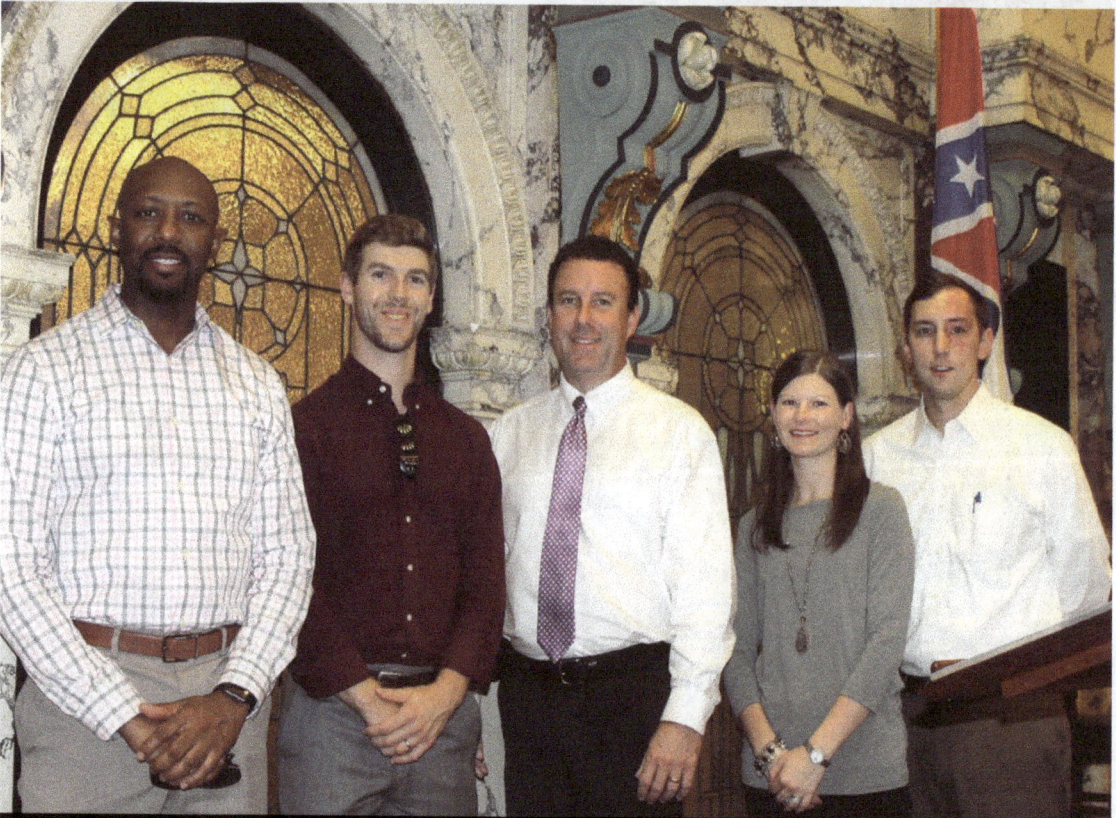

2018, Leadership Optometry class at the Mississippi Capitol. L-R: Eric Johnson OD, Chris Herring OD, Senator David Parker OD, Mandi Smith OD, Bran Dawson OD.

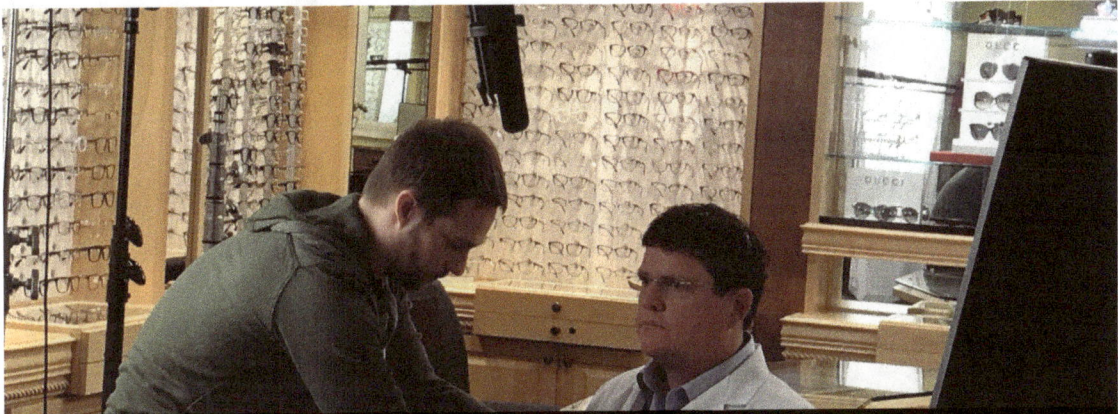

2018 Marketing and Branding campaign with Adaptive Branding. Jacob Ivey, OD gets mic'ed in preparation for filming.

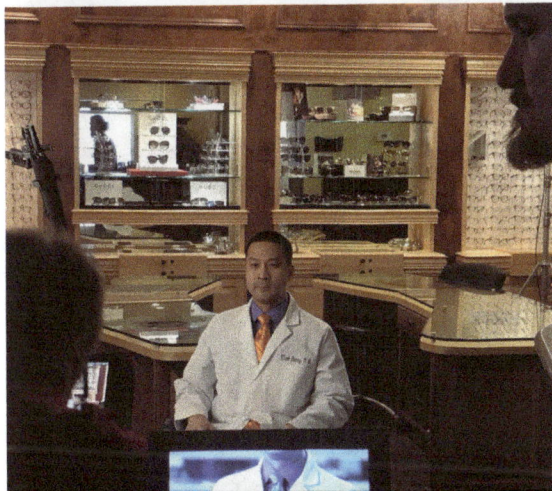

2018 Marketing and Branding campaign with Adaptive Branding. Filming Minh Duong, OD.

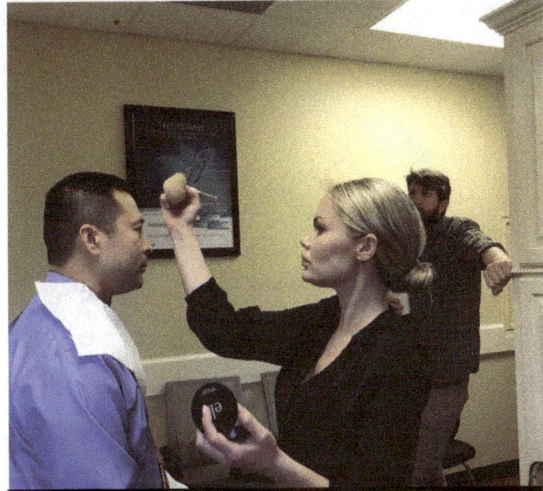

Marketing and Branding campaign with Adaptive Branding. Minh Duong, OD gets powdered in preparation for filming.

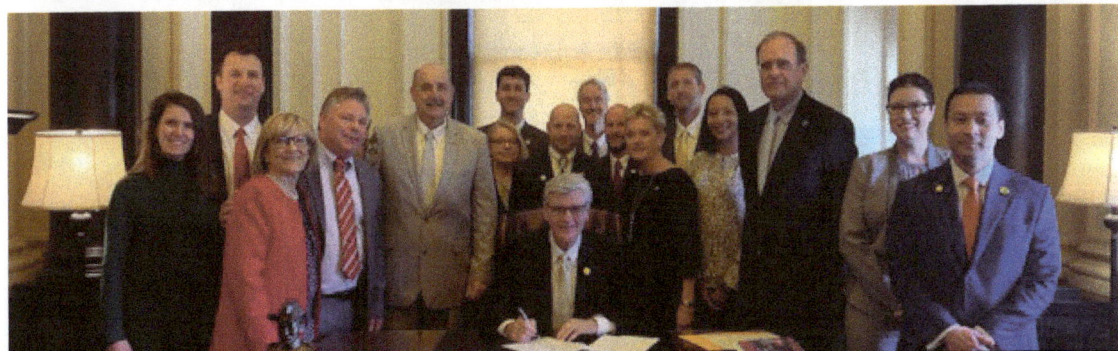

2019 Children's Vision bill signed by Governor Phil Bryant. L-R behind Governor Bryant: Megan Lott, OD, Blake Bell, Linda Ross Aldy, CAE, Representative Rob Roberson, Cynthia Huff, Representative Richard Bennett, Patti Permenter, Ed.D, Ryan Wally, OD, Greg Loose, OD, Steven Reed, OD, Evan Davis, OD, Amy Crigler, OD, Senator Chris Caughman, Kimberly Ragan, OD, Secretary of State Delbert Hosemann, Sarah Link, CAE, Minh Duong, OD

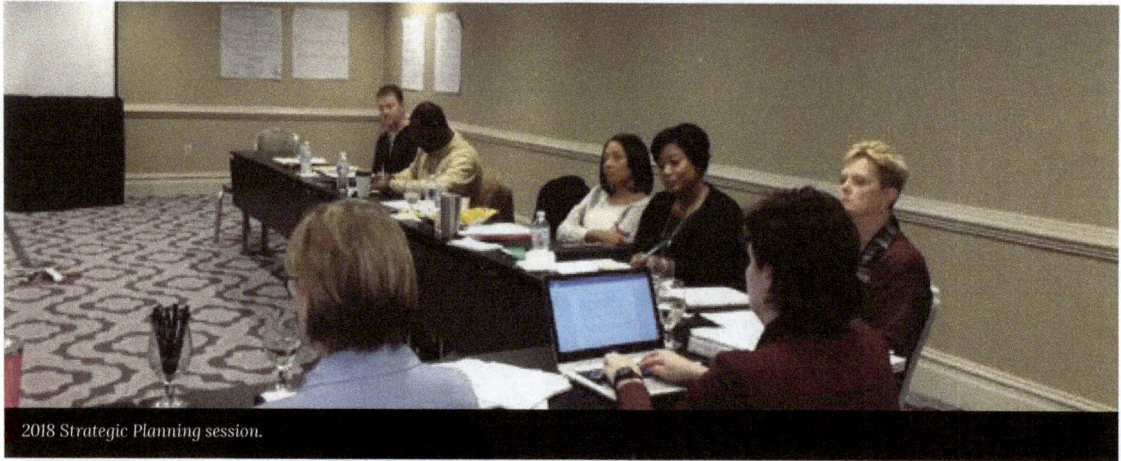

2018 Strategic Planning session.

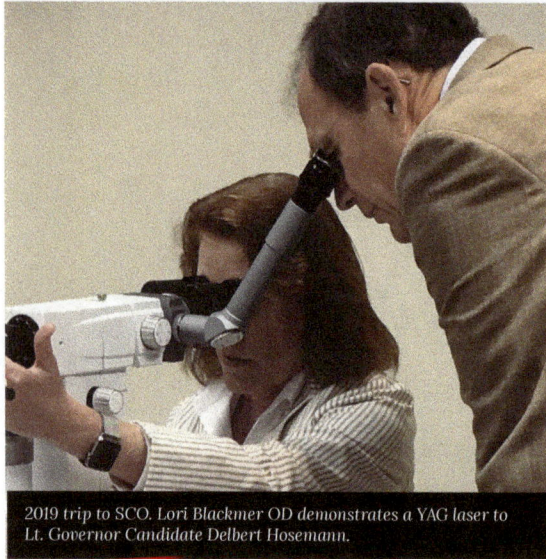

2019 trip to SCO. Lori Blackmer OD demonstrates a YAG laser to Lt. Governor Candidate Delbert Hosemann.

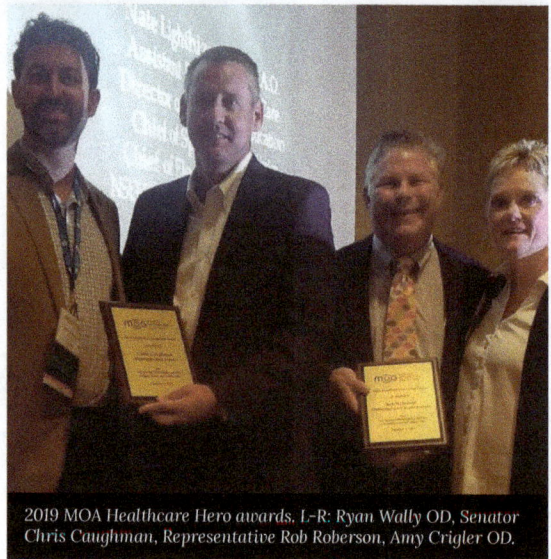

2019 MOA Healthcare Hero awards. L-R: Ryan Wally OD, Senator Chris Caughman, Representative Rob Roberson, Amy Crigler OD.

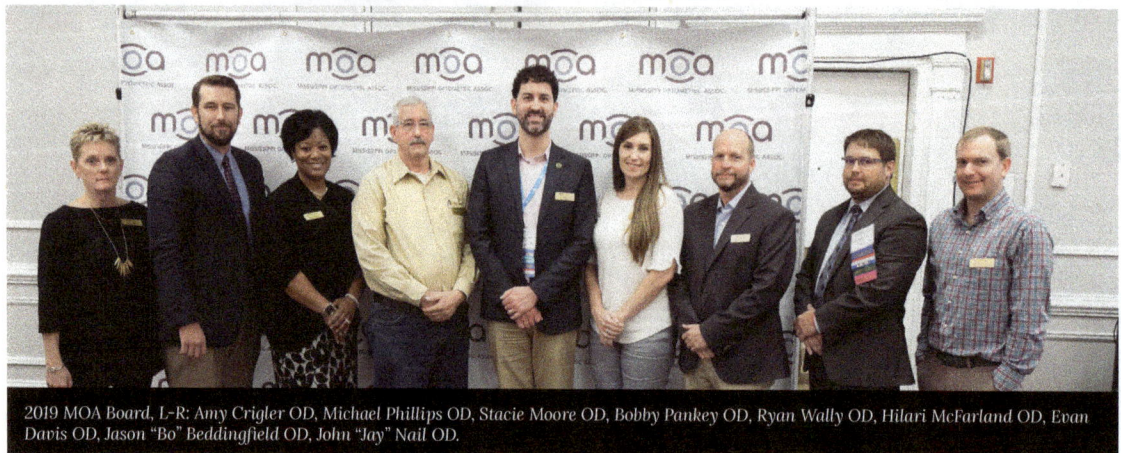

2019 MOA Board, L-R: Amy Crigler OD, Michael Phillips OD, Stacie Moore OD, Bobby Pankey OD, Ryan Wally OD, Hilari McFarland OD, Evan Davis OD, Jason "Bo" Beddingfield OD, John "Jay" Nail OD.

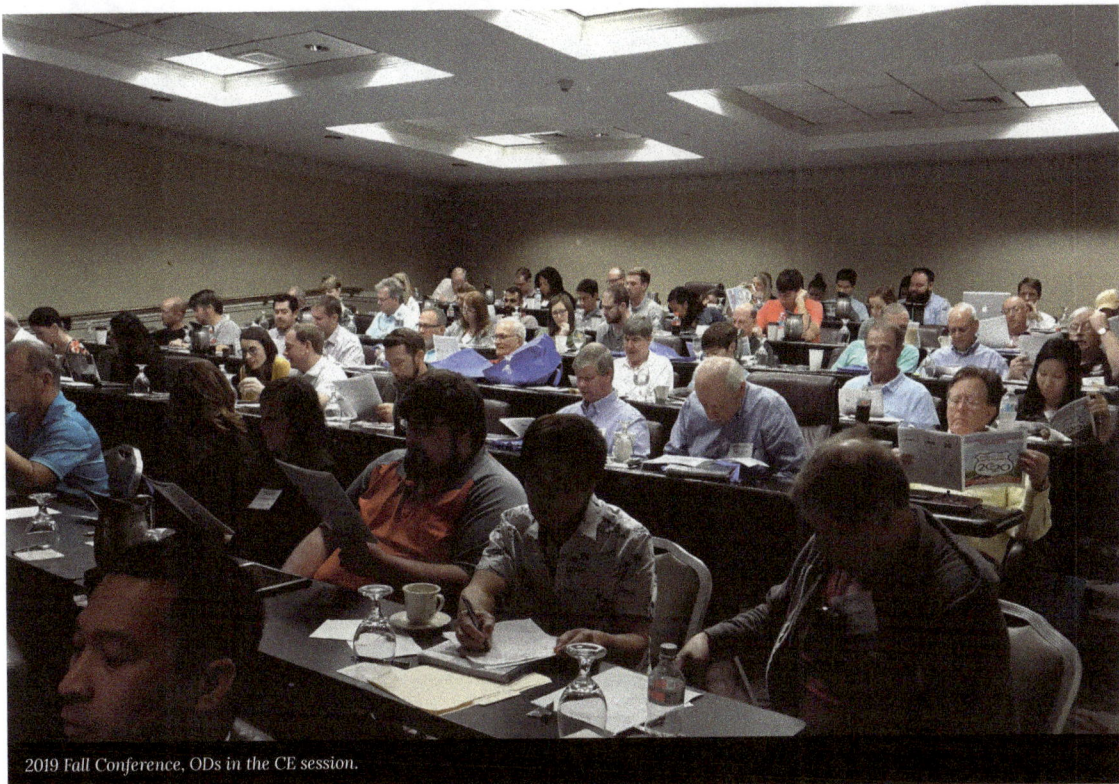

2019 Fall Conference, ODs in the CE session.

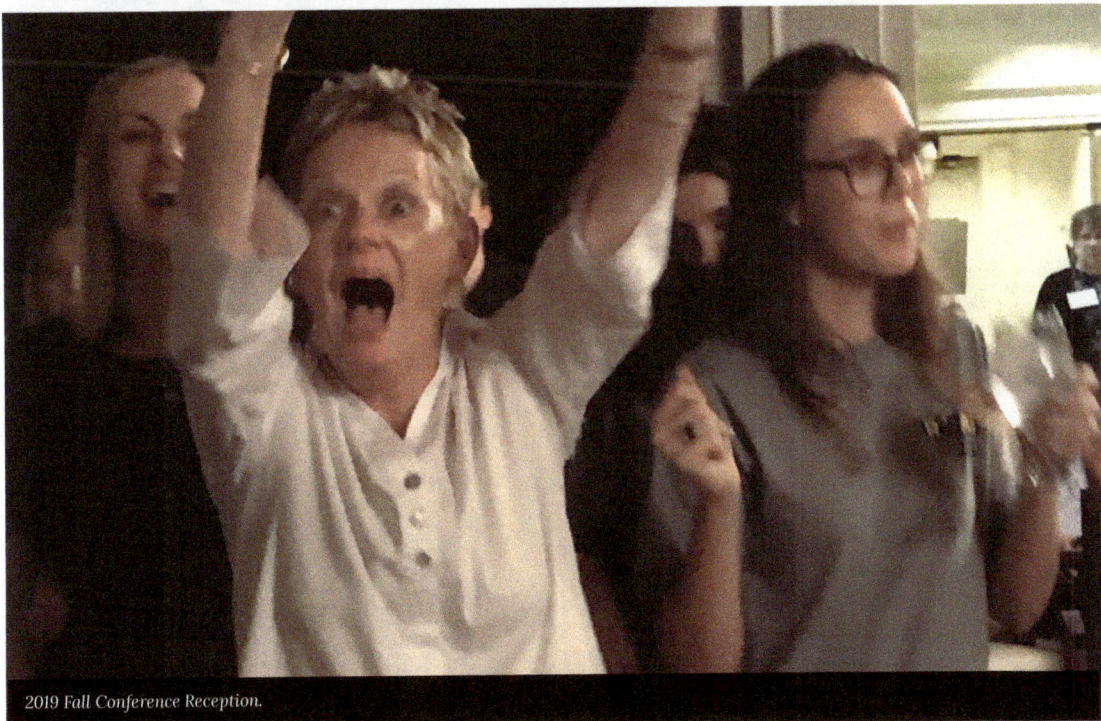

2019 Fall Conference Reception.

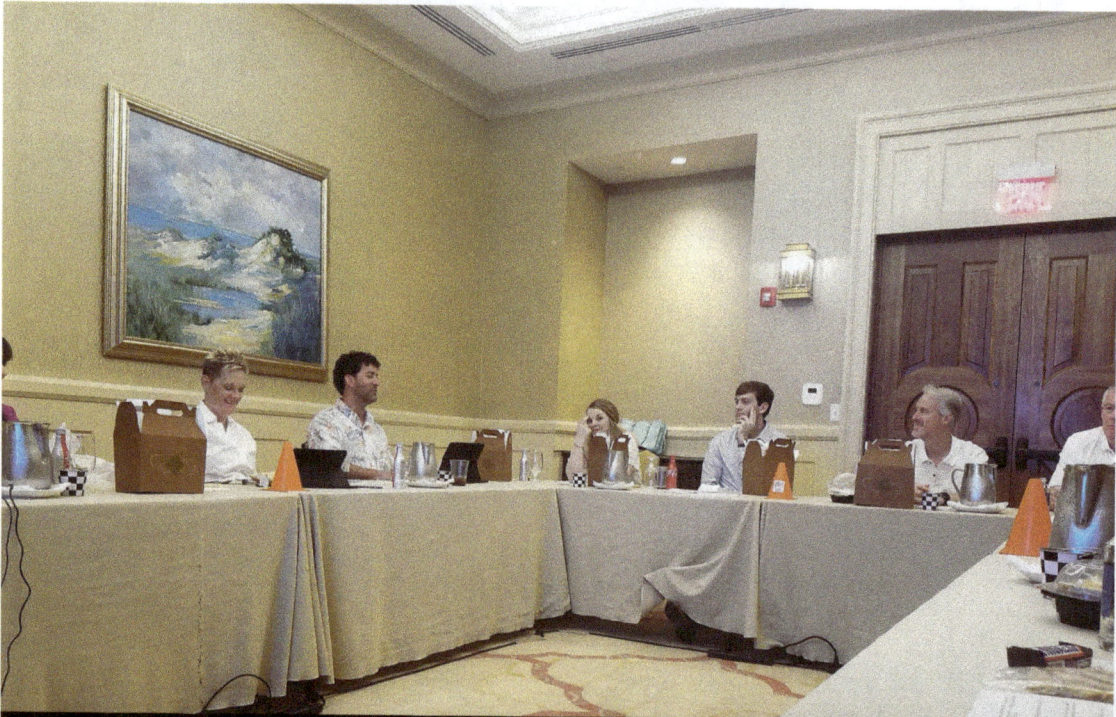

2019 Leadership Optometry class. L-R: Roya Attar OD, Amy Crigler OD, Ryan Wally OD, Kelli Mullen OD, R. Slater Smith OD, Steven Reed OD, Bill Reynolds OD (AOA Trustee).

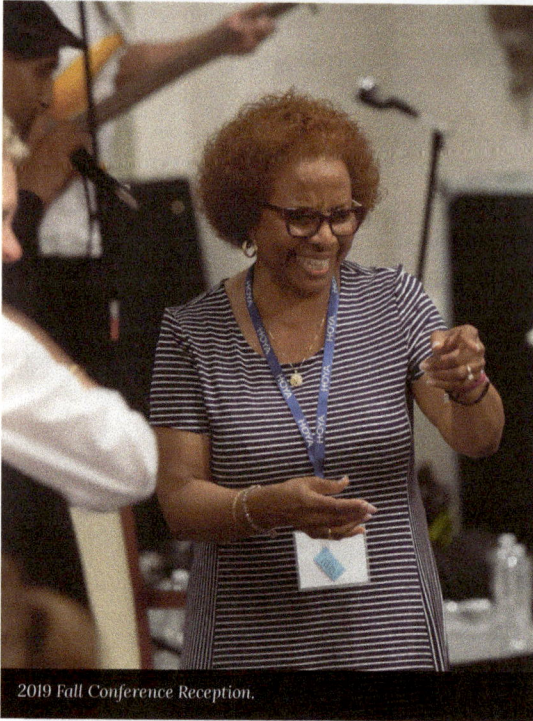

2019 Fall Conference Reception.

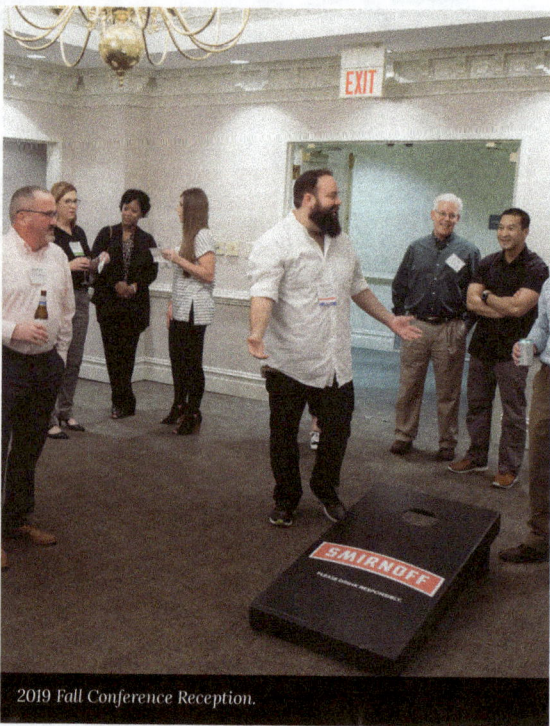

2019 Fall Conference Reception.

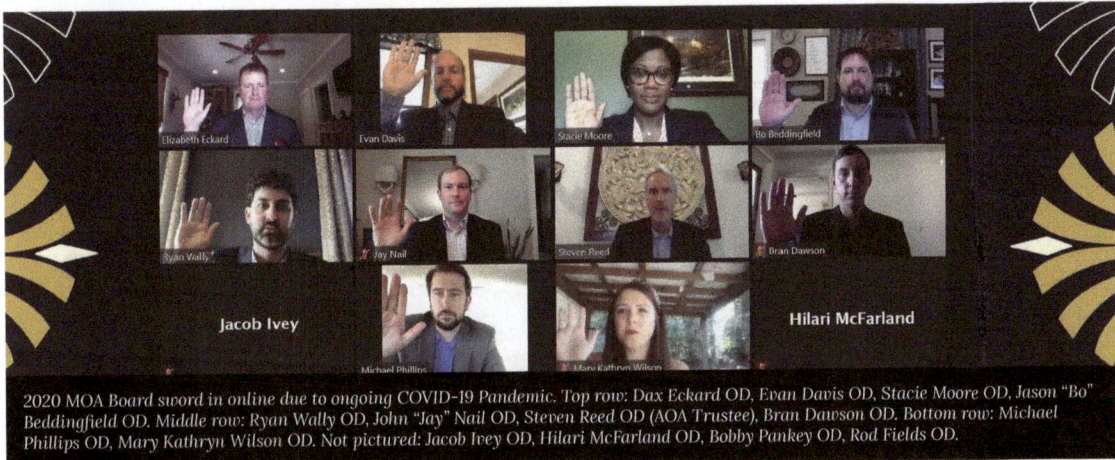

2020 MOA Board sword in online due to ongoing COVID-19 Pandemic. Top row: Dax Eckard OD, Evan Davis OD, Stacie Moore OD, Jason "Bo" Beddingfield OD. Middle row: Ryan Wally OD, John "Jay" Nail OD, Steven Reed OD (AOA Trustee), Bran Dawson OD. Bottom row: Michael Phillips OD, Mary Kathryn Wilson OD. Not pictured: Jacob Ivey OD, Hilari McFarland OD, Bobby Pankey OD, Rod Fields OD.

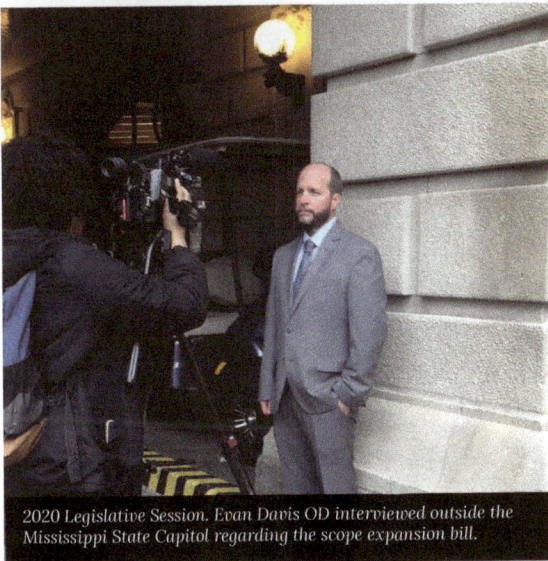

2020 Legislative Session. Evan Davis OD interviewed outside the Mississippi State Capitol regarding the scope expansion bill.

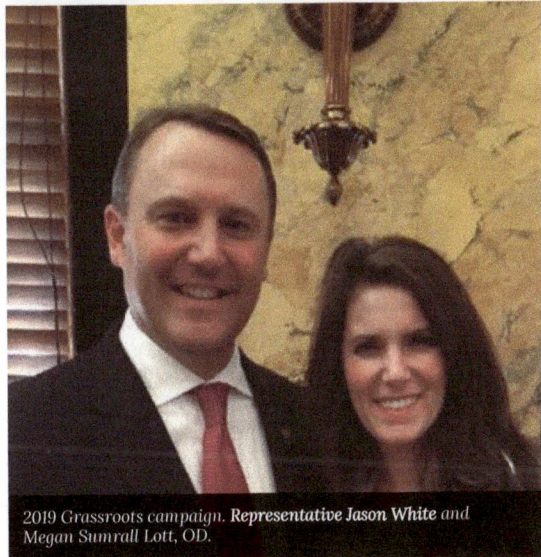

2019 Grassroots campaign. **Representative Jason White** and Megan Sumrall Lott, OD.

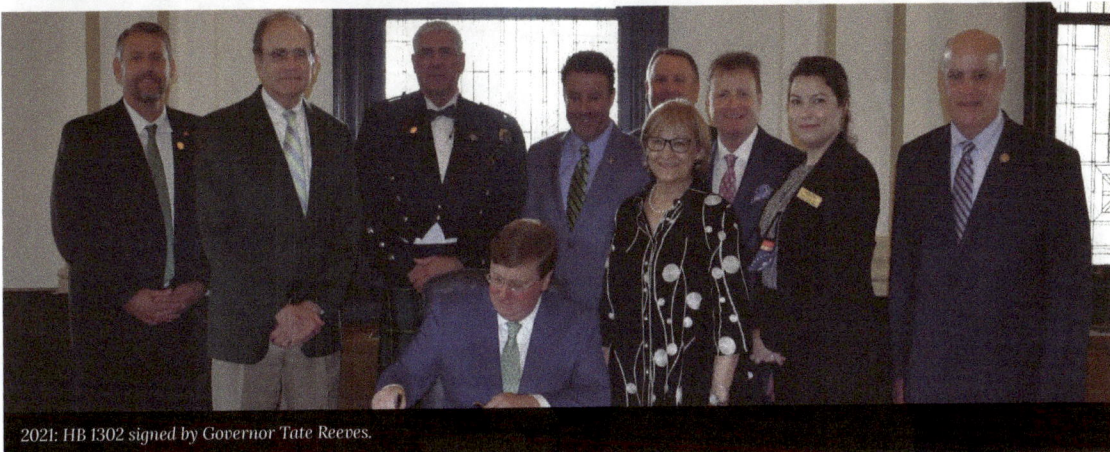

2021: HB 1302 signed by Governor Tate Reeves.

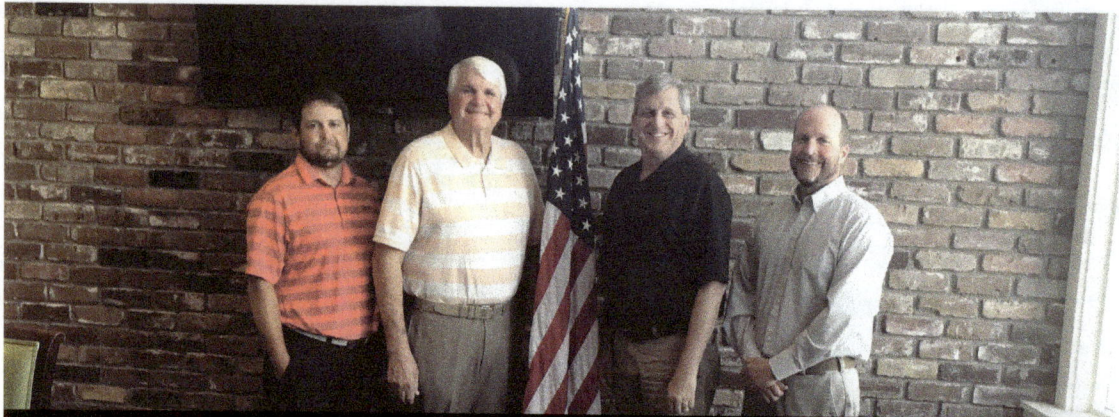

2019 Grassroots campaign. Jason "Bo" Beddingfield OD, Representative Gary Staples, Representative Donnie Scoggins, Evan Davis OD.

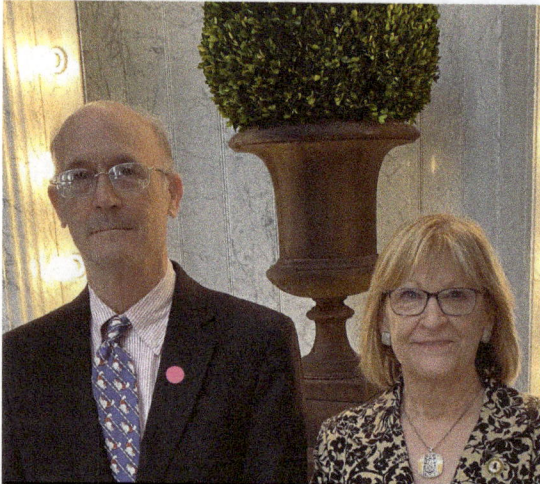

2021 Legislative Session. Senator Hob Bryan and Linda Ross Aldy, CAE on the day HB 1302 passed out of Senate.

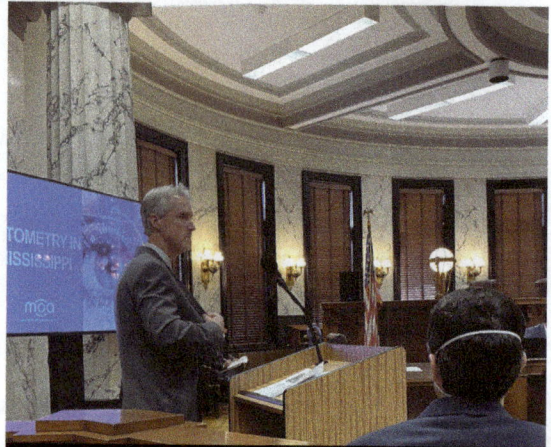

October 2020. Steven Reed, OD testifies in front of Mississippi Senate Public Health Committee, while Senator David Parker, OD observes from the background. Face masks are being worn due to the COVID-19 pandemic.

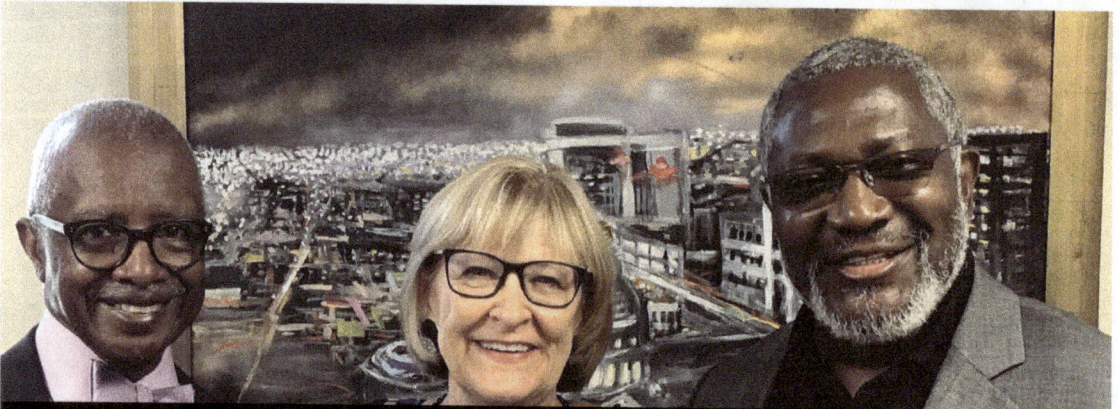

2019 Grassroots Campaign. Senator Hillman Frazier, Linda Ross Aldy CAE, Senator John Horhn.

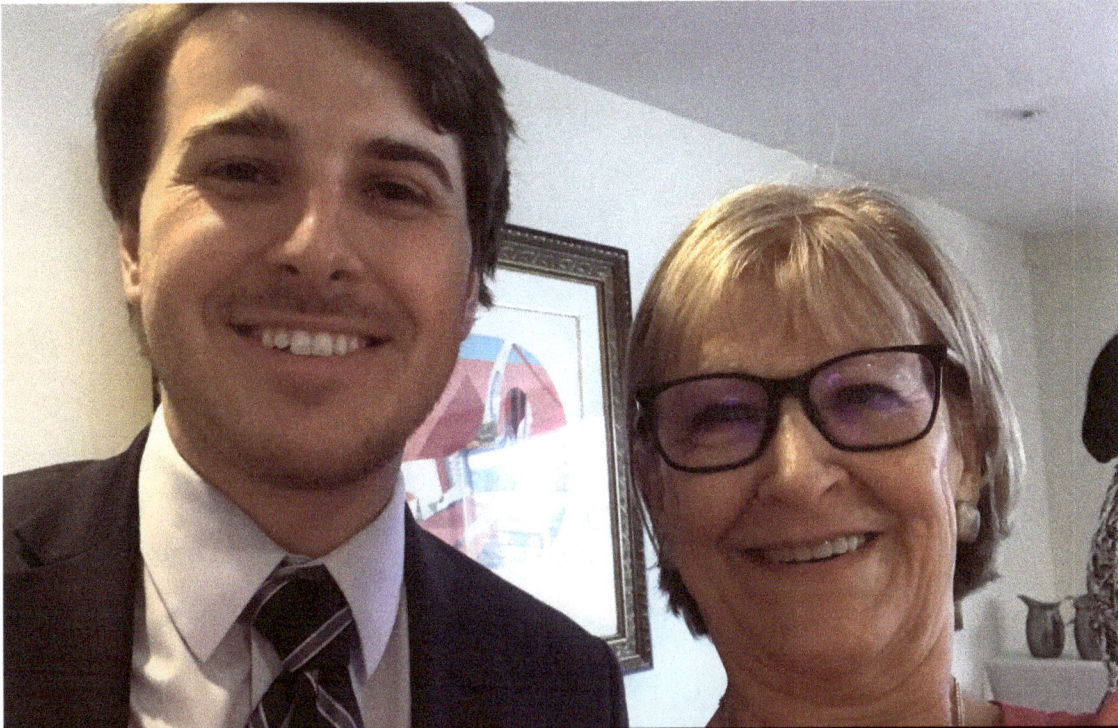

2019 Grassroots Campaign. Representative Kent McCarty and Linda Ross Aldy, CAE.

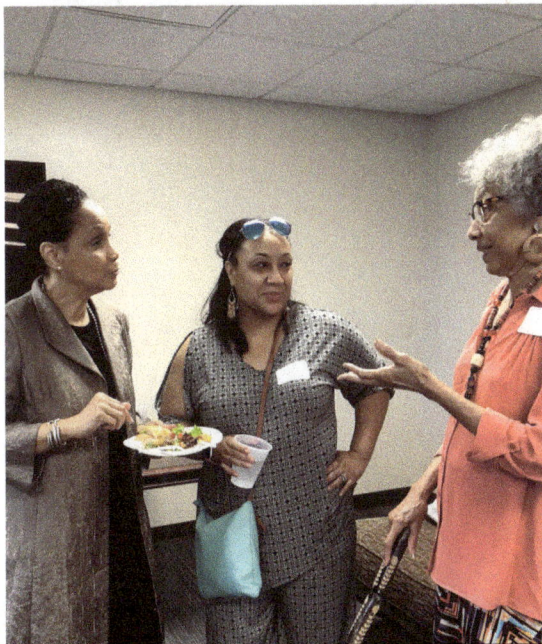

2019 Grassroots Campaign. Monique Carr, OD and Representative Alyce Griffin Clarke.

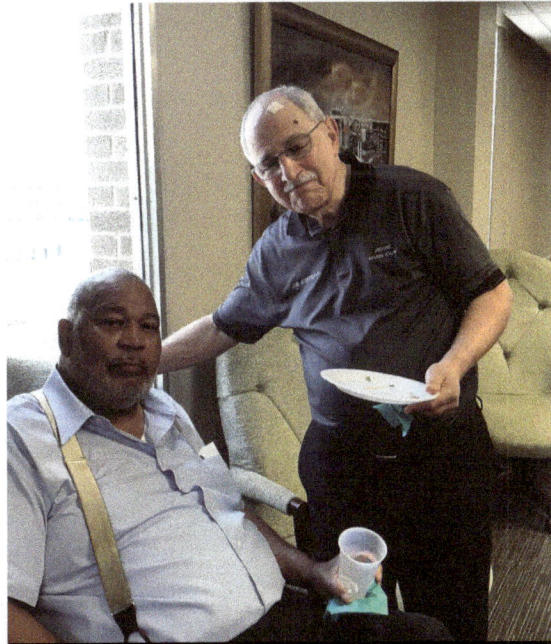

2019 Grassroots Campaign. Representative Willie Bailey and Joe Joseph, OD.

CHAPTER 03

The Mississippi State Board of Optometry

The Mississippi Legislature passed the state's first optometry practice act in 1920 (See Appendix, attachment 2). The new law created the State Board of Examiners in Optometry and allowed the Board to issue licenses to those in the existing practice of "optometry" whether they had formal training or not. There were four main functions of the Board: (1) develop and issue rules and regulations for the practice of optometry; (2) examination of applicants for licensure; (3) issue licenses to practice; and (4) enforcement of the Optometry Practice Act.

One hundred and thirty-seven licenses were issued on February 7 and 8, 1920. In July, another ten licenses were issued.

After searching for the Board's records, the first Board minutes found were recorded June 10, 1927. The meeting of the Board was held at the Capitol in Jackson. The minutes of that June 10 meeting recorded that there were three applicants for initial licensure, and three Mississippi optometrists were reviewed regarding the establishment of temporary offices. After thorough investigations, the cases were dismissed. The meeting also included several request for reciprocity to practice in Mississippi, and all were denied. During the early years, there were many requests for reciprocity; some were granted and some denied. Reciprocity became a frequent issue with the board.

During the June 10 meeting, the Board passed a resolution to pay the Board secretary $25 per month. Elections of officers were held and all current officers were re-elected. The records reflect that the Board usually met twice a year to ensure enforcement of the Optometry Law, to examine candidates, to issue licenses, and to elect officers. The meetings were held in Jackson in several venues; the State Office Building, the King Edward Hotel, the Walthall Hotel, and the Heidelberg Hotel.

At the July 8, 1929, meeting a motion was made and passed to notify all licensees that the $2 renewal fee was due and if not paid, their certificate of licensure would be revoked. True to their word, the Board revoked thirty-seven licenses January 13, 1930.

The minutes of January 11, 1932, recorded the election of officers and two applicants for examination and licensure. One applicant did not meet the educational requirements, and the other was from Memphis who asked to practice one day each week in Holly Springs. The Board rejected the reciprocity request. The Board contended it would not grant any more reciprocity certificates unless the applicant moved into Mississippi and established a permanent office in the state and became a citizen of Mississippi.

In January 1935, the Board, acting under the optometry law, issued the following agreement with an optometrist in Jackson:

1. Will not accept employment with a corporation
2. Will not advertise
3. Will not solicit business from house to house.
4. Will have no more than three locations.
5. Will practice under the Code of Ethics of Optometry

At the time the subjects on the examination included anatomy, practical theory of optometry, physiological optics, pathology and physiology, and demonstration of lens neutralization.

At the January 1939 meeting, the Board fixed the salary of the Board Secretary at $100 per year, and to cover any secretarial expenses. The Board also considered a violation of an optometrist delegating exams to unqualified staff. According to the Board minutes, "The accused optometrist promised to be good."

The Board decided at the September 18 meeting to draft a resolution commending Dr. H.C. Green, Clarksdale, for his service as president. Shortly thereafter, Dr. Green, after attending an MOA meeting in Oxford, was returning to Clarksdale and was killed when his plane crashed on takeoff. The resolution was later presented to Mrs. Green.

After World War II, the GI Bill of Rights provided educational opportunity for military veterans. Consequently, there was a considerable increase in the number of students entering optometry schools across the country. From 1947 to 1951, the Mississippi Board examined ninety-one candidates for licensure. Most passed the exam, and those who failed were eligible for re-examination.

The Board agreed during the January 1950 meeting that "a person not serve on both the MOA board and the state board." Also, the president of the Board was to inform the MOA of actions taken by the Board. One candidate passed the exam, but had to wait until his *twenty-first birthday* to be licensed.

A complaint was filed at the January 1951 meeting against an optometrist in Lucedale who was practicing without a license. After investigation, the Board authorized the board attorney, Richard Billups Jr., to prepare and file injunction proceedings. There was also a complaint filed by the MOA regarding an optometrist aiding and abetting Sears, Roebuck and Company in the unlawful practice of optometry.

A special meeting of the Board was held June 12, 1951, to consider recommendations made by the MOA. The Board approved the following actions:

1. The secretary of the Mississippi State Board of Optometry is to mail a copy of the court opinion and final decree regarding the Sears case to each optometrist in Mississippi. This mailing was to include copies of the Rules and Regulations promulgated by the Board. And to prepare a news release regarding the Sears case.
2. The Board authorized Mr. Billups to write each company or corporation advising them of the decision of the court and give them notice to stop the unlawful practice of optometry or face an injunction suit to stop such unlawful practice.

The first African American optometrist licensed in Mississippi, Dr. David W. White, Jackson, took and passed the board exam at the Woolfolk Building on July 9, 1951.

Following a request made by the MOA at the January 1954 meeting, an injunction was filed against three optometrists practicing in a corporate environment. At the July meeting, the Board considered a request by the MOA for revision of the Board Rules and Regulations. Discussion of the request was deferred pending the outcome of other matters. MOA also requested authorization to file injunction proceedings against the Mississippi State Board of Health to stop discrimination against optometry. The request was deferred for further study.

At this juncture, it is important to note that the State Board and the MOA had together become much more assertive in its actions against the unlawful practice of optometry and discrimination by governmental agencies. In Dr. Eric Muir's 1981 paper (see Appendix) he attributed this, in large part, to the legal wisdom of Richard Billups who was serving as legal counsel for both the MOA and the State Board.

In January 1957 the Board voted to proceed with an injunction against the Mississippi State Board of Health for discrimination against optometry. The Board also increased the penalty for delinquent payment of relicensing fees to $15. Twelve licenses were revoked for nonpayment at the next meeting. The Board also ruled "any agreement between a lay organization and a professional man, whereby the lay organization advocates and steers patients to that man would be considered by the Board to be unprofessional and unethical conduct." Billups rides again.

A joint meeting of the State Board and the MOA was held in Jackson at the Sun-n-Sand Motor Hotel in September 1961. The State Board announced it was investigating an optometrist for dispensing hearing aids. The optometrist was to be visited and counseled by a State Board member. Also, there was a discussion regarding Southern Regional Education Board scholarships available to Mississippi students.

Nota bene: The minutes of the State Board meetings from 1961 to 1987 are not to be found.

In August 1987, Medicare determined that doctors of optometry are now considered physicians for Medicare purposes.

The March 9, 1988, Board meeting was held at the Sheraton Hotel in Jackson, and was open to the public. The new Board legal counsel, Mark Chinn, raised issues regarding the administration of Board business practices. After discussion the following administration directives were adopted:

1. Board counsel shall be responsible for drafting meeting minutes to be approved by the Board.
2. Board counsel to make available the minutes within a reasonable time and be available for inspection.
3. Board to retain minutes.
4. Board counsel to prepare a handbook for each Board member with the Mississippi Optometry Act, Board regulations, and administrative procedure.
5. Board counsel to prepare the meeting agenda at the direction of the Board secretary.
6. All communications with Board members are to be copied to each member including third-party correspondence.
7. Board counsel shall submit statement for services monthly.
8. Board counsel to add a paralegal to take on more administrative responsibilities of the Board.

Dr. John Mohr, Pearl, reported on the Senate Judiciary Committee's action regarding responsibilities that the legislature may place on the Board relative to the use of pharmaceutical agents. (Side note: In November 2019, Dr. Mohr, the second oldest active practitioner in the U.S., retired at age 91).

The Board also unanimously voted to direct counsel to prepare a legal opinion regarding reimbursement for services of optometrists by the Mississippi Medicaid Commission. The Board also discussed recent publicity regarding fee sharing for patients referred from optometrists to ophthalmologists.
At the November 1988 meeting, it was reported that the Medicaid Commission had submitted the matter of reimbursement to the state attorney general for an opinion.

In January 1989, the Board tabled a motion to require the National Board exam. In June, the attorney general found it was not appropriate for the Medicaid Commission to deny reimbursement to optometrists. The Medicaid Commission was given to July 1, 1989, to adopt a new policy. Noteworthy: The Board voted to require National Board of Examiners of Optometry (NBEO) examinations. Also at the June meeting, the Board filed an injunction regarding the illegal practice of unlicensed persons substituting optometrists' prescriptions. Application forms for candidates for licensure were updated. The Board voted to join New Mexico in objecting to Eyeglass II ruling of the Federal Trade Commission.

In July, the Board voted to delay implementing NBEO exam for one year to give adequate advance warning to applicants. A new pharmacology exam was approved to give to approximately two hundred existing optometrists. By unanimous vote, the Board approved the NBEO's Treatment and Management of Ocular Disease (TMOD) examination for licensure effective July 1990.

At the November 1989 meeting there were more complaints to consider. An injunction was filed against Optical Warehouse for violating the Optometric Practice Act. The Board voted to require each applicant for licensure to bring their own patient for the practical exam. At the January 1990 meeting the Board voted to publish updated Rules and Regulations.

In June 1990, the Board considered the required Sunset Review scheduled for 1991, directed legal counsel to investigate the illegal practice of optometry by corporations, to develop recommendations for enforcement, and to investigate violations of the contact lens law. In September the Board continued to investigate advertising by optometrists; and reported that "Eyeglass II" ruling had been overturned.

On October 13, 1991, the Board agreed to meet with the State Board of Medical

Licensure to discuss the problems regarding the interrelationship between optometry and ophthalmology. At the November meeting the Board considered allowing practice management courses for continuing education credit, and to require CPR every two years instead of every year. On November 21, the optometry board attended a meeting with the State Board of Medical Licensure that was presided over by Attorney General Mike Moore. Both boards agreed to appoint an *ad hoc committee* to study the relationship between the two professions.

At the October 1992 meeting, the Board ruled all phases of the NBEO would be required. Each Phase I applicant to be tested on Mississippi Optometry Law, is to include test on Board Rules and Regulations. There was a discussion of upcoming legislation and re-licensure fee increases. The Board voted to allow four hours of practice management, and permitted two hours of correspondence courses for continuing education purposes.

At the November 6, 1993, the Board secretary appealed for the hiring of a CPA to meet state financial requirements. The secretary also reported a lack of funds to meet the current responsibilities of the Board. Fortunately, the MOA supported an annual fee increase of $300 for license renewals.

In January 1994, the Board discussed the introduction of legislation by MOA to authorize the use of pharmaceutical agents for the treatment of eye disease and eye injury. During the legislative session HB 1859 was passed authorizing optometrists to use therapeutic pharmaceutical agents (TPA).

A special meeting was called May 2, to pass a regulation setting forth the educational and clinical requirements for certification to use pharmaceutical agents to treat eye disease and eye injury as set forth in HB 1859.

At the June 10 meeting, the Board adopted the didactic and clinical requirements of HB 1859 that authorized the use of therapeutic pharmaceutical agents. The Board also met with officers of the MOA to discuss the implementation of HB 1859. Applicants for authority to treat ocular disease and eye injury must pass the TMOD examination given by the National Board of Examiners of Optometry. At the January 1995 meeting the MOA presented codes for Medicare reimbursement. The Board directed legal counsel to write Medicare for immediate approval. In February, Rule 38 was amended: (1) Successful passage of the TMOD given by the National Board and/or other appropriate examination approved by the Mississippi State Board of Optometry; and (2), All therapeutically certified optometrists are required to obtain twenty hours of continuing education each year for a long as they are in practice, eight of those hours shall consist of therapeutic subject matter.

During the July 1996 meeting, the Board discussed possible actions to be taken when an optometrist fails to inform the Board where their office is located. The Board also considered procedures for foreign applicants desiring to obtain a Mississippi license. A rule change was suggested requiring all *new licensees* to be TPA certified.

In January 1997 one license was revoked, and "full-time" practice was defined as requiring twenty hours of work each week for the purpose of taking the Phase II exam. In February, the Board deleted the waiver of continuing education for persons over the age of 65. At the June meeting, the Board approved four hours of continuing education by correspondence, and agreed to hire a professional secretary to assist the Board secretary. The contract for legal services was continued with Chinn & Associates. In July, Board counsel was directed to contact the attorney general's office regarding the obtaining of contact lenses by mail order.

At the January 1998 meeting, the Board questioned the Mississippi student contract rule requiring graduates to practice in Mississippi or pay back the stipend. The Board directed counsel to research the matter. A draft of the state PEER Review committee was reviewed at the July 1998 meeting. The report included the following background information: "In recent years with the arrival of contact lenses and easier to use diagnostic drugs, optometrists have sought to change their profession from prescribing and selling glasses to a full-fledged healthcare profession. This has resulted in states expanding the scope of practice by authorizing optometrists' use of diagnostic and therapeutic pharmaceutical agents. Since 1989 all states have authorized optometrists' use of diagnostic pharmaceutical agents (DPA's), which is a limited category of drugs used to enable a more thorough eye examination. This was followed by optometrists seeking the privilege of using topical or systemic drugs for the treatment of eye disease or injury (with) therapeutic pharmaceutical agents (TPA's). As of 1997, all states allowed optometrists the use of TPA's. However, significant variance existed regarding the conditions that optometrists can treat and the drugs they use."

The PEER Review committee recommended: "The Board of Optometry and the Board of Medical Licensure should jointly develop written recommendations for presentation to the Legislature in January 1999. These recommendations should specify how the Boards plan to work together to: (a) determine the causes for the shortage of optometrists and ophthalmologists in Mississippi; and (b) develop a plan for providing eye care services to meet the state's needs."
At this juncture it is evident that the Rules and Regulations governing the practice of optometry had come a long way since 1920. The State Board's responsibility to regulate the profession of optometry was playing an extremely important role in the advancement of the profession. It might be noted that at almost every meeting the Board considered complaints concerning licensed optometrists. When they found it necessary, the Board took appropriate

action, including license suspension.

At the March 2000 meeting, Beverly Limbaugh was hired as the Executive Assistant. The Board also went on record to oppose establishment of the American Board of Optometric Practice (ABOP). Also in 2000, the Federal Drug Administration seized contact lenses sold illegally in Brookhaven and McComb. In 2000, there were two hundred and sixteen optometrists licensed to practice in Mississippi.

In 2001, the Board eliminated the Phase II examination. *The Clarion-Ledger* and others were issued subpoena for accepting illegal advertisements by optometrists. A letter of warning was sent to various entities regarding the unlawful dispensing of contact lenses. Three optometrists were assessed $500 for rule violations.

The Board announced at the January 2003 meeting that optometrists are to have TPA certification by 2006. The annual report to the governor included issues such as standardization of licensure, the illegal sale of contact lenses, corporate practice violations, and continuity of patient care. At the November meeting, the Board reviewed the Mississippi Supreme Court ruling that "Board rules & regulations must be reasonable, shall not be capricious or arbitrary, be within the Board's power and *not* violate a party's constitutional rights."

A special meeting was called in March 2005 for approval of a continuing education course: "Oral Medications for Primary Care." Governor Haley Barbour signed SB 2682 which allowed the use of oral medications. In June, Rule 6.2 regarding oral medications was filed with the Secretary of State's office. The Board agreed to extend continuing education requirements for those optometrists affected by Hurricane Katrina.

In June 2006, the Board met in court before Judge Denise Owens to defend the adoption of Rule 12.5 requiring that all optometrists with a current license and no TPA or DPA certification, and those with DPA certification only, must meet the education requirements to obtain their TPA certification by December 31, 2006. Subsequently, the court ruled that Rule 12.5 as promulgated by the Mississippi Board of Optometry was invalid. In November, Rule 12.5 was suspended.

During the January 2007 meeting the Board discussed holding district meetings to review the Rules and Regulations. It was announced that two hundred ninety-five optometrists were licensed to practice in Mississippi. At the June meeting, it was announced that the governor had signed SB 2682 that gave prescriptive authority to Mississippi optometrists for schedule IV & V controlled oral medications as they pertain to the treatment of eye disease and injury. In November Dr. Janice Jacobs, Ocean Springs, became the first woman to be appointed to the State Board. CPT codes were approved for low vision and vision therapy.

In June 2008, the Board challenged Walmart for violations of the Optometry Act, and approved Optometric Education Tracker. In November, a letter was received from Walmart addressing the concerns of the Board.

In January 2009, the Board considered a proposal regarding CPT codes from the Mississippi Optometric Association. The Board responded to the November letter from Walmart. Four optometrists were fined for rule violations. In June, Dr. Dewey Handy, Jackson, became the first African American to be appointed to the State Board.

During the March 2011 meeting, the Board issued a cease-and-desist letter to an optical company in Grenada for violating the Optometry Law. It was announced that three hundred and thirty optometrists were licensed to practice in Mississippi.

In January 2013, the Board issued a $500 fine for unprofessional conduct, administered a Rules and Regulations exam to five applicants, and addressed the illegal sale of contact lenses. An undercover operation by the attorney general's office, working with the Mississippi Board of Optometry, resulted in six arrests on allegations of unauthorized fitting of contact lenses.

At the June 2014 meeting, the Board reviewed a complaint against an optometrist for allegedly having a relationship with a married patient. No action was taken. The Board also reviewed a case regarding an optometrist seeing patients while "high" on drugs. The Board counseled the optometrist. The Board formally issued the following mission statement: "The mission of the Mississippi Board of Optometry is to appropriately license and renew licenses of optometrists in the state, and to regulate the practice of optometry by concentrating on enforcing the Practice Act and the Rules & Regulations to protect the citizens of Mississippi."

It was reported that 2015 began with three hundred and sixty-six licensed optometrists, and the year ended with three hundred and eighty-eight licensed optometrists. In 2016, Beverly Limbaugh's title was changed to executive secretary, and a new website for licensure renewal was launched. A memo was sent to all Mississippi optometrists regarding the improper use of the title of "Board Certified." An Attorney General's opinion regarding the unlawful practice of online eye exams and the online sale of contact lenses was issued. During the July 2017 meeting, the Board suspended an optometrist's license for drug abuse. In December, due to the many new regulations and the extremely detailed issue of "fair play" required of regulatory boards, the Board held an orientation class on regulatory authority and procedure.

Notably, as the general public became more aware of the laws governing the responsibilities of healthcare providers, there were increased complaints filed against healthcare practitioners. Optometry was no exception to legal liability. This resulted in an increasing number of complaints received and investigated by the State Board.

Over the past one hundred years, the Board of Optometry has played a vital role in the progress of the profession, dealing with complaints, sanctioning those in violation, giving exams, supporting legislation to expand the scope of practice, and protecting the right to practice optometry in Mississippi. The men and women who have, and are, serving on the Board have rendered a great service to the profession and to the public. They are to be commended for their time and effort.

CHAPTER 04

Optometry in Mississippi: A personal history

My maternal grandfather, James H. Edgar, grew up in Sharp County, Arkansas, near Hardy. In 1907, at age 17, he traveled to St. Louis, Missouri, and worked in a shoe factory and studied watchmaking, or horology. Later, he graduated in 1916 from Needles Institute of Optometry, a one-year optometry program in Kansas City. Dr. William Brag Needles later moved his school to Chicago and merged with Northern Illinois College of Optometry, now known as Illinois College of Optometry.

Grandfather was drafted into the army just as the United States was entering World War 1 in 1917. He completed basic training at Jefferson Barracks Military Post located on the Mississippi River about 10 miles south of St. Louis. As his division was about to embark to France, he was hospitalized with pneumonia, which caused him to miss the train trek to New York to ship out to France. After recovery, he was discharged from the army in 1917. He traveled back to Arkansas riding a mule, and along the way he worked for farmers for food and a place to sleep.

He then set up practice as an optometrist in Little Rock where he soon met the woman who would be my grandmother, Fannie Lee Weir, who worked in a department store. Not long after their marriage in 1919, they moved to Hattiesburg, Mississippi. Hattiesburg was a major railroad hub (giving the city the moniker "Hub City"). Grandfather Edgar contracted with a railroad company to repair and maintain all of their clocks and watches. At that time the railways ran by the clock and the telegraph. Although Grandfather Edgar was busy maintaining and repairing clocks and watches, he did practice optometry. He eventually opened his own jewelry store, Edgar Jewelry.

Mississippi passed its Optometry Act in 1920, the forty-seventh state to do so. In just two days after enactment, one hundred and thirty-seven individuals were licensed. Grandfather Jim Edgar held license number 46. The new law "grandfathered in" all the individuals who called themselves optometrist, optician, or refracting optician; some, such as my grandfather, had formal training, some had taken correspondence courses, and some just fit glasses. Notably, a number of those first licensed optometrist had children that also eventually became optometrists in Mississippi.

My mother, Nell W. Edgar, was born in 1920. Grandfather's jewelry store/optometry practice was successful; however, in 1929 the store caught fire and burned to the ground. This was the beginning of the Great Depression and the insurance company with which he held an insurance policy had declared bankruptcy a few days before the fire. Without insurance to cover the loss, Grandfather Edgar was unable to continue operation of the jewelry store. He turned to the full-time practice of optometry.

Throughout the Great Depression, the Edgar family was fortunate to make ends meet. Grandfather had twenty-five acres on which to raise cows, chickens, and to grow a garden. The home and acreages were located on 25th Avenue where the current University of Southern Mississippi women's softball field is located.

As the United States began to gear up for entry into World War II, Camp Shelby, located just south of Hattiesburg, would become one of the largest army basic training camps in the country. Obviously the army trainees had to have good eyesight to qualify on the firing range. Since there were no optometrists commissioned in the army, the Defense Department contracted with Grandfather Edgar to examine and prescribe spectacles -- two pair of glasses and gas mask inserts -- for those soldiers failing the vision screening test.

As a result of the government contract, Grandfather Edgar was very busy; seeing private patients in the morning and examining soldiers in the afternoon and early evening. Meanwhile, my mother, Nell Edgar, graduated from Southern College of Optometry (SCO) in 1943 and joined her father in his practice, lightening his workload.

My father, Nash Cochran from Fort Myers, Florida, entered SCO in 1941, and that is where he met my mother. With the bombing of Pearl Harbor on December 7, 1941, my father, along with most of the SCO students, enrolled in military service. After basic training at Fort Oglethorpe in Georgia, he was assigned to teach army air corps bombardiers how to use the newly developed Norden bombsight.

The army released father to finish optometry school and he graduated in early 1944. Nell Edgar and Nash Cochran married in the fall of 1944 and began a partnership practice in Kosciusko. On October 5, 1945, I, William E. Cochran, was born and entered the world of optometry and so far it has been an incredible journey.

My earliest recollection of optometry came from going with my parents and grandfather when they attended educational and business meetings of the

Mississippi Optometric Association. At the time there were no requirements for continuing education for optometrist. Nevertheless, many optometrists who had a great interest in advancing the profession participated in the educational presentations.

At these meetings, usually at the Heidelberg Hotel on Capitol Street in Jackson, my Grandmother Edgar would "babysit" me while mother, father, Grandfather Edgar, and my mother's brother, Frank Edgar, Hattiesburg, attended the educational and business sessions. In those days it was not unusual for children to roam the hotel and even stroll along Capitol Street. I was no exception.

I had my first encounter with optometric education at about age six. It has been told that I was bored with walking around the hotel and "crashed" one of the educational sessions instructed by A. M. Skeffington, O.D. Dr. Skeffington was from Oklahoma and had cofounded the Optometric Extension Program, a successful monthly subscription study series that included vision development, vision therapy, and practice management. He was also famous for his three-piece suits and spats (to the younger generation, spats were worn above one's shoes). He lectured extensively around the country and traveled only by train. Most of his presentations centered on vision development and vision therapy. During this particular session "Skeff," as he was fondly known, presented a discussion of accommodation and convergence, including accommodative rock therapy. It seems that I had climbed up on my mother's lap and had listened intently to the presentation. A few days later, my parents took me to a movie in Kosciusko. Father had parked the car across the street in a parking lot that was outlined with sizable rocks. As we crossed the street, I looked at one of the rocks and asked the question, "Is that an accommodative rock?"

As I grew older I remember hearing about subjects that were of concern to the members of the Association, continuing education, obstruction by ophthalmology, school screening, and ethical practice, etc. In the late 1950s my mother chaired the Association's Ethics Committee, and I remember she had to reprimand a member of the Association for giving out pencils with the optometrist's name and address imprinted on it. Advertising in any form was considered unethical.

In 1977 the United States Supreme Court (Bates v. Arizona State Bar Association) ruled that the prohibition of advertising by lawyers (by inference other professions: medical doctors, dentists, and optometrists) violated the First Amendment upholding the right of lawyers to advertise their services. This was a hard pill to swallow for the members of the Association after years of struggle to prohibit advertising by optometrists.

Through the years I attended the Association's annual conventions with my parents. The convention was usually held in Jackson and Primos Cafe, located on Capitol Street, had the best chocolate brownies with sugar on the bottom. To this day when I am in Jackson, I still get them from Primos in the famous purple box.

When the State Board of Examiners began requiring continuing education for optometrists in the late 1950s, the Association moved the annual education conference to the University of Mississippi. After attending one of those meetings, mother brought me an Ole Miss football jersey that I wore with great pride. Most of the optometrists in the state obtained their annual education requirements at the Ole Miss conference.

I attended my first American Optometric Association Convention at age 12. My mother was a delegate and we drove to Washington, D.C., in the summer of 1958. This was before air-conditioned cars; it was hot. What a great adventure for me, as I had only been out of Mississippi a few times to visit my paternal grandparents in Florida. The nation's capital was quite an educational experience; visiting Mt. Vernon, the Jefferson Memorial, the White House, the Washington Monument, and the National Military Cemetery. My favorite was the Smithsonian Museum of History.

In the early 1960s, the Association's convention moved to the Mississippi Gulf Coast. The beach and wonderful seafood made it a great venue for a convention. I can remember hearing about comedian Brother Dave Gardner at Gus Stevens Supper Club.

As late as the 1960s Mississippi had not yet repealed the National Prohibition Act of 1919. Indeed, Mississippi was the last state to do so. Yet in most parts of the state one could purchase bonded alcohol from "bootleggers," especially in the Delta and on the Gulf Coast where liquor stores abounded even though the sale of liquor was illegal. Nevertheless, if you could put money on the counter, you could be accommodated.

I pass this history along simply because imbibing alcohol in the hospitality rooms at the Association's convention was part and parcel of the meeting. Great fellowship and camaraderie brought the members of the Association together, which enhanced the desire to advance the profession.

After attending my freshman year at the University of Southern Mississippi, I worked at Central Optical Company in Jackson during the summer of 1964. Working at the wholesale lab was a great experience for me because it included rotation through the processes of marking lenses, generating, cutting and edging, mounting lenses in frames, and mailing the finished product to optometrists around the state. That summer the Association convention was held in Greenville. Of course, Central Optical had a hospitality room. Bob Bowman, manager of the Jackson lab, allowed his son, Bob Jr., and me to tend the bar. What fun! Of course, we only mixed and served drinks.

I began my formal optometric education at SCO in 1965. It was great to develop lifelong friendships with Mississippi students: Watts Davis, Bernard Ellis, Jim Coe, W.C. Maples, Earl Malone, and Paul Clark. After graduating in 1968 (my class was the next-to-last class that had a three-year curriculum before the establishment of the four-year curriculum) Carolyn Euart and I were married in June 1968, and I entered military service in October.

The Army Medical Service Corps was also a learning experience for me. Optometrists had finally been given direct commissions as second lieutenants. During the Vietnam War the army temporally promoted optometrists to captain upon entrance to active duty. The army allowed optometrists to use diagnostic pharmaceutical agents. Many optometrists who served during the Vietnam War soon joined the national movement to expand the scope of practice. By the way, Col. John Leddy, originally from McComb, Mississippi, served as the commanding officer of the Optometry Section of the Army Medical Service Corps. He was a 1956 graduate of SCO, and after retiring from military service, served on the SCO Board of Trustees.

After being honorably discharged from the army in 1970, I entered private practice in Kosciusko with my mother. The Mississippi Optometric Association was just beginning its effort to expand the scope of practice that resulted in a battle royal with ophthalmology. Dr. Eric Muir details that effort in his 1981 paper (see Appendix).

In 1974 the Association hired its first executive director. Up until that time, the Association depended upon the Association's elected secretary to keep minutes and manage the affairs of the Association. Helen St. Clair was hired as the second executive director in 1976. One could write for a long time about the impact that Helen had on the profession, both in the MOA and AOA, and in the IAOE, the International Association of Optometric Executives. She quietly guided the Association through the many legislative battles that led to the expansion of the scope of practice. She was a mentor to me, and to all the Association's leadership teams over the next two decades. In fact, Helen encouraged me to apply for the position of president of SCO. Had she not made that suggestion I would most likely still be in Kosciusko. Her legacy continues to this day.

During the 1970s, Mississippi optometry focused its attention on implementing legislation expanding the scope of practice. Passing such legislation required the involvement of all the optometrists practicing in the state. It also required leadership. Those in leadership positions that led the early legislative effort included: L. B. Adkins, W. F. Clark, W. M. Dickerson, Paul A. Doherty, Rayford Edgar, William. J. Goyer, W. S. Harper, John J. Hora, Paul Lycette, Horace L. May, Eric Muir, Andy Reese, Walt Simpson, R.G. Stribling, Roland Stevens, and Charles P. Tillman, just to name a few. At the time Richard Billups Jr was the Association's attorney. Billups had more to do with advancing the profession of optometry in Mississippi than any other single person. His involvement is presented in Dr. Muir's paper.

I became a member of the Association in 1970. Probably because I had grown up as an O.C. (optometrist's child), the officers and directors knew me; therefore, I was elected to the board of directors in 1973. To prepare for the coming effort to expand the scope of practice, the Association sponsored a transcript quality course in pharmacology in 1976. The course was offered by SCO and a large percentage of Mississippi optometrists took the course and passed the examinations. Shortly after the final examination, the Association's annual education meeting took place at Ole Miss. After studying pharmacology for weeks there was a collective sigh of relief at the meeting.

Shortly after my father, Nash Cochran, was appointed to the State Board of Examiners I received a call from him. It seems he was assigned the optics portion of the Board examination. He asked if I had any old optics exams saved from my student days at SCO. I said, "yes," and sent him copies of several exams. A few days later he called and said, "OK, you s.o.b., where are the answers?"

In 1977 I was elected president of the Association. The Association was in the thick of the legislative battle with ophthalmology to pass legislation to allow optometrists to use diagnostic pharmaceutical agents. Finally, after consistent efforts on the part of the Association, the Mississippi Legislature passed HB 475 in 1982 that allowed optometrists to use pharmaceutical agents for diagnostic purposes.

But the battle was not over. For several more years, ophthalmology continued to introduce legislation to repeal the new optometry law, but to no avail. The Association continued its efforts to pass legislation allowing optometrists to practice to the full extent of their education and training.

Later as president of Southern College of Optometry, it was an honor and pleasure to testify several times before the various committees of the Mississippi Legislature regarding the current education and training required for the doctor of optometry degree.

It is difficult to fully explain the many years of effort by the Mississippi Optometric Association to enhance the scope of practice. Needless to say without the Association the practice of modern optometry in Mississippi would not exist.

I must say that the Mississippi Optometric Association played a significant role in my life, as well as in my career. I will be forever thankful. The lesson learned: "Eternal vigilance is the price of liberty."

Appendix

1. Mississippi Optical Society
2. Original Law, Rules & Regulations Enacted on 1920
3. MOA Annual Convention Program, 1943
4. MOA Articles of Incorporation - 1947
5. Plain Talk Editorial, Mississippi Optometrist, 1950
6. 1957 MOA Officers
7. 1960 MOA Officers and Members
8. SCO Mississippi Club, 1967
9. MOA Annual Convention Program, 1973
10. Photos from 1981 Strategic Planning Session, 1981
11. President's Message, Dr. Jim Brownlee, 1982
12. Save Your Vision Week, Proclamation, 1989
13. Senate Bill 2682, Oral Medication Bill
14. Past Presidents of the Mississippi Optometric Association
15. Photo of SB 2682 being signed, 2005
16. Photo of HB 1302 being signed, 2021

OPTICAL JOURNAL
November 1, 1906 (8:19)

the matter
the profes-
ississippi, I
attention of
icient num-
e an effort
need to be
rill be glad
r with any
rest mani-
RIGGS.
Optician.

MISSISSIPPI OPTICAL SOCIETY.

This new society held a fall gathering at the Edwards House, Jackson, Miss., on October 24 last. The meeting was large and enthusiastic. The day was spent in discussing matters pertaining to the benefit of this influential organization. Among the regulations passed was the following, which will be of interest to the people of the State, assuring them better work:

"Resolved, That all applicants for admission to this society be examined upon the following subjects: The anatomy of the eye, refraction, optics and practical experience."

This society has had such a large growth that it feels the time at hand when it can make admission into its membership a thorough test of the educational qualities of the applicant. Plans were also brought forth looking toward the passing of a State law regulating the practice of optometry similar to that in force in California and Minnesota.

After business was over the following educational program was carried out: "Anatomy of the Eye," F. W. Queen; "Muscular Anomalies," E. R. von Seuter; "Light and Lenses," Dr. A. I. Orr; "Correcting Astigmatism," L. M. Guess; "Benefits of Organization," M. F. Fritz; "Modern Optician," T. L. Mitchell.

The next meeting will be held at Tattiesburg on the second Tuesday and Wednesday of next May.

1. Mississippi Optical Society

OPTOMETRY
IN
MISSISSIPPI

Law, Rules, Regulations

❦

Enacted 1920

Issued by
**Mississippi State Board
of Examiners in
Optometry**

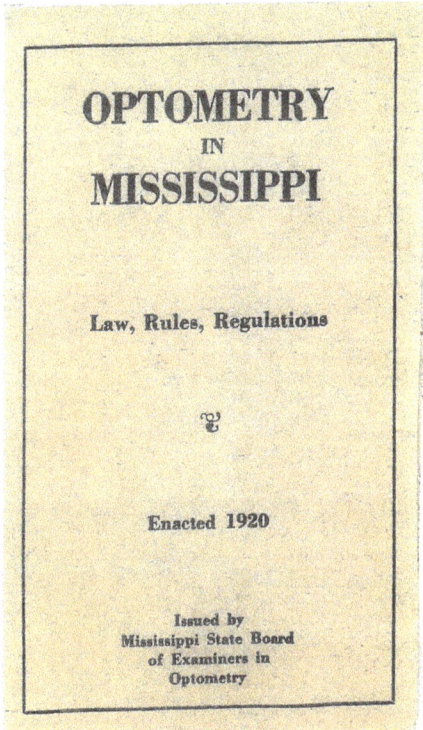

Mississippi Code 1930 Annotated

Chapter 140 as amended by Chapter 326 of 1932
(Vol. 2)

Be It Enacted by the Legislature of the State of
Mississippi:

Optometry—Practice of, Defined

Paragraph 5652. The practice of optometry is defined to be the application of optical principles through technical methods and devices in the examination of human eyes for the purpose of ascertaining departures from the normal, measuring their functional powers and adapting optical accessories for the aid thereof.

(6124a; 1920 ch. 217)

Who May Practice—Examination and License

Paragraph 5653. It shall not be lawful for any person in this state to engage in the practice of optometry or to hold himself out as a practitioner of optometry, or attempt to determine by an examination of the eyes the kind of glasses needed by any person, or to hold himself out as able to examine the eyes of any person for the purpose of fitting the same with glasses, excepting those hereinafter exempted, unless he has first fulfilled the requirements of this chapter and has received a certificate of licensure from the State Board of Optometry created by this Chapter, nor shall it be lawful for any person in this State to represent that he is the lawful holder of a certificate of licensure such as provided for in this Chapter, when in fact he is not such lawful holder, or to impersonate any licensed practitioner of optometry or to fail to register the certificate as provided by law.

(6124b; 1920 ch. 217)

Penalty for Violations of this Chapter

Paragraph 5654. Any person violating the provisions of this Chapter shall be guilty of a misdemeanor and, upon conviction, for his first offense shall be fined not more than five hundred dollars at the discretion of the court, and upon conviction for a second or later offense shall be fined not less than five hundred dollars, nor more than one thousand dollars or imprisoned not less than six months nor more than one year at the discretion of the court.

(6124c; 1920 ch. 217)

Board of Optometry—Appointment of—Qualifications

Paragraph 5655. The Governor, with the advice and consent of the Senate, shall appoint a State Board of Optometry consisting of five persons, citizens of Mississippi, each of whom shall be a nonmedical man or woman, actually engaged in the practice of optometry for five years next preceding his appointment.

No person so appointed shall be a stockholder in or member of the faculty, or of the board of trustees of any school of optometry, or serve to exceed two terms.

Vacancies on said Board shall be filled by appointment by the Governor.

(6124d; 1920 ch. 217)

Organization of Board—Officers—Meeting and Powers

Paragraph 5656. The State Board of Optometry shall organize by the election from its members of a President and a Secretary, who shall hold their respective offices for one year.

It shall hold regular meetings for examination, beginning on the second week of January and July of each year, and additional meetings at such times and such places as it shall determine, not to exceed one every three months, but the July meeting shall be held in the City of Jackson.

A majority of the Board shall constitute a quorum but a less number may adjourn from time to time.

The Board shall make such rules and regulations as may be necessary to carry out the provisions of this Chapter; provided, however, that it shall require the concurrence of a majority of the members of the Board to grant or revoke a license.

(6124e; 120 ch. 217)

Secretary of Board—Bond and Oath of Office Required

Paragraph 5657. Before entering upon the discharge of the duties of his office the Secretary of the State Board of Optometry shall give a bond to the State, to be approved by the Board, in the sum of two thousand dollars conditioned for the faithful discharge of the duties of his office. The premium for such bond to be paid from the funds paid into the State Treasury by the Secretary of the Board.

Such bond with the approval of the Board, and oath of office indorsed thereon, shall be deposited with the Secretary of State and kept in his office. Each month all moneys received by the Secretary shall be paid by him into the State Treasury to the credit of a fund for the use of the State Board of Optometry.

(6124f; 1920 ch. 217)

Compensation of Secretary and Members—How Paid

Paragraph 5658. Each member of the State Board of Optometry shall receive five dollars for each day actually employed in the discharge of his official duties, and his necessary expenses incurred.

The Secretary shall receive an annual salary to be fixed by the Board, and his necessary expenses incurred in the discharge of his official duties.

The compensation and expenses of the Secretary and members of the Board and the expenses of the Board necessary in carrying out the provisions of this chapter, shall be paid from the fund in the State Treasury for use of the Board on the requisition signed by the President and the Secretary of the Board and the warrant of the Auditor of the State; provided, however, the said compensation and expenses shall not exceed the amount paid into the State Treasury under the provisions of this chapter.

(6124g; 1920 ch. 217)

Board to Have Seal and Keep Records of All Business

Paragraph 5659. The State Board of Optometry shall have an official seal and shall keep a record of its proceedings, a register of persons registered as optometrists and register of licenses by it revoked.

Its records shall be open to public inspection, and it shall keep on file all examination papers for a period of ninety days after such examination. A transcript of an entry in such records, certified by the Secretary under the seal of the Board, shall be evidence of the facts therein stated. The Board shall annually, on or before the first day of January, make a report to the Governor of all its official acts during the preceding year, and of its receipts and disbursements and a full and complete report of the conditions of optometry in this state.

(6124h; 1920 ch. 217)

Examination—Who Required to Take—Qualifications

Paragraph 5660. Any person over the age of twenty-one years, of good moral character, and who has graduated from a High School or Preparatory School affiliated with and recognized by a

2. Original Law, Rules & Regulations Enacted on 1920 (pg. 1)

State University, and who has graduated from a reputable School or College of Optometry maintaining a two-year course in optometry, each session seven months in length, and offering a course of a standard equivalent to that required by the Federal Board of Vocational Training, shall be entitled to stand the examination for license to practice optometry in Mississippi. The Examining Board of Optometry shall keep on file a list of schools or colleges of optometry which are recognized by said Board and which give a course in optometry equivalent to the requirements or standard heretofore specified.

The examination to practice optometry shall consist of tests in practical, theoretical and physiological optics, in theoretical and practical optometry and in anatomy and physiology of the eye and in pathology as applied to optometry.

(6124i; 1920 ch. 217)

Applicants Examination, Failure—Re-Examination— Displaying Certificate—Peddling—Temporary Offices—Fees

Paragraph 5661. Every person desiring to be licensed as in this chapter provided, shall file with the Secretary of said Board upon appropriate blank to be furnished by said Secretary an application, verified by oath, setting forth the facts which entitle the applicant to examination and licensure under the provisions of this chapter. The said Board shall hold at least two examinations each year. In case of failure at any standard examination the applicant, after the expiration of six months and within two years, shall have the privilege of a second examination by the Board without the payment of an additional fee. In case of failure at any limited examination, the applicant shall have the privilege of continuing the practice of optometry and of taking a second examination without the payment of an additional fee. Every applicant who shall pass the standard examination, and who shall otherwise comply with the provisions of this chapter, shall receive from the said Board under its seal a certificate of licensure entitling him to practice optometry in this State, which certificate shall be duly registered in a record book to be properly kept by the Secretary of the Board for that purpose, which shall be open to public inspection, and a duly certified copy of said record shall be received as evidence in all courts of this State in the trial of any case. Each person to whom a certificate shall be issued by said Board shall keep said certificate displayed in a conspicuous place in office or place of business wherein said person shall practice optometry, together with the photograph

of said person attached to the lower righthand corner of said certificate and shall whenever required exhibit the said certificate to any member or agent of said Board.

Peddling from door to door, or the establishment of temporary offices is especially forbidden under penalty of revocation of said certificate by said Board. Whenever any person shall practice optometry outside of or away from his office or place of business he shall deliver to each person, fitted with glasses by him, a certificate signed by him wherein he shall set forth the amounts charged, his postoffice address and the number of his certificate. Each person to whom a certificate has been issued by said Board shall before practicing under the same register said certificate in the office of the Clerk of the Circuit Court in each county wherein he proposes to practice optometry, and shall pay therefor such fee as may be lawfully chargeable for such registry. The clerk of the Circuit Court in each county shall keep a certificate registration book wherein he shall promptly register each certificate for which the fee is paid.

(6124j; 1920 ch. 217)

Fee for Certificates and Renewal—Revocation of License

Paragraph 5662. Said Board shall charge the following fees for examinations, registrations and renewals of certificates. The sum of twenty-five dollars for a standard examination, and twenty-five dollars for a limited examination. Every registered optometrist who desires to continue the practice of optometry shall, annually, on or before the first day of January, pay to the Secretary of the Board a renewal registration fee of five dollars, for which he shall receive a renewal of his certificate.

In case of neglect to pay the renewal registration fee herein specified, the Board may revoke such certificate and the holder thereof may be reinstated by complying with the conditions specified in this chapter. But no certificate or permit shall be revoked without giving sixty days' notice to the delinquent, who, within such period shall have the right of renewal of such certificate on payment of the renewal fee with a penalty of five dollars, provided, that retirement from practice for a period not exceeding five years shall not deprive the holder of said certificate of the right to renew his certificate on the payment of all lapsed fees.

The Board shall adopt a seal and certificate of suitable design and shall have an office at Jackson, in this State, where examinations may be held and where all its permanent records shall be kept,

Paragraph 5663. The Board shall refuse to grant a certificate of licensure to any applicant and may cancel, revoke or suspend the operation of any certificate if it granted for any or all of the following reasons, to-wit: The conviction of a crime involving moral turpitude, habitual intemperance in the use of ardent spirits, or stimulants, narcotics or any other substance which impairs the intellect and judgment to such an extent as to incapacitate for the performance of the duties of an optometrist. The certificate of licensure of any person convicted of a violation of Second Section of this chapter shall be ipso facto revoked.

Any person who is a holder of a certificate of licensure or who is an applicant for examination for a certificate of licensure, against whom is preferred any charges, shall be furnished with a copy of the complaint and shall have a hearing before the Board, at which hearing he may be represented by counsel. At such hearing witnesses may be examined for and against the accused respecting the said charges, which examination shall be conducted in the manner usually followed in the taking of testimony before commissions in this State. The suspension of a certificate of licensure, by reason of the use of stimulants or narcotics, may be removed when the holder thereof shall have been adjudged by the said Board to be cured and capable of practicing optometry.

(6124l; 1920 ch. 217)

Certificates of Other States—When and How Recognized

Paragraph 5664. An applicant for a certificate of licensure who has been examined by the State Board of another State which, through reciprocity, similarly accredits the holder of a certificate issued by the Board of this State to the full privileges of practice within such State shall, on the payment of a fee of twenty-five dollars to the said Board and on filing in the office of the Board a true and attested copy of the said license, certified by the President or Secretary of the State Board issuing the same and showing also that the standard

License Does Not Entitle to Treat with Drugs or Medicines

Paragraph 5665. Nothing in this chapter shall be construed as conferring on the holder of any certificate of licensure issued by said Board the title of doctor, oculist, ophthalmologist, or any other word or abbreviation indicating that he is engaged in the practice of medicine or surgery, or the treatment or the diagnosis of diseases of, or injuries to the human eye, or the right to use drugs or medicines in any forms for the treatment or examination of the human eye.

(6124n; 1920 ch. 217)

Physicians, Druggists and Merchants May Sell Spectacles

Paragraph 5666. The provisions of this chapter shall not apply to physicians or surgeons practicing under authority of licenses issued under the laws of this State for the practice of medicine or surgery. And provided that this chapter shall not prohibit merchants and druggists who are actually engaged in this state from selling and assisting purchasers in fitting spectacles and eyeglasses in their place of business at time of sale.

(6124o; 1920 ch. 217)

2. Original Law, Rules & Regulations Enacted on 1920 (pg. 2)

THIRTY-EIGHTH

ANNUAL CONVENTION

OF THE

MISSISSIPPI

OPTOMETRIC ASSOCIATION

★

HEIDELBERG HOTEL

JACKSON, MISSISSIPPI

SUNDAY, APRIL 18, 1943

PROGRAM
★

9 A. M. to 10 A. M.—Registration

10 A. M.—Address by President
Dr. R. H. Marsh.

10:15 A. M.—Dr. D. H. Orkin—
Organizational Advancement
Student Procurement and General
Discussion on Subject.

11:00 A. M.—Dr. J. W. Rothchild—
Public Relations and General
Discussion.

Noon.

1:30 P. M.—Dr. A. A. Schamber
Ethics and Economics and General
Discussion.

2:00 P. M.—Dr. L. O. Embry—
Subject to be announced.

2:30 P. M.—Business Session
Report of Dr. D. H. Orkin,
Secretary-Treasurer.
Adoption of New Constitution and
By-Laws.
Election of Officers.

3. MOA Annual Convention Program, 1943

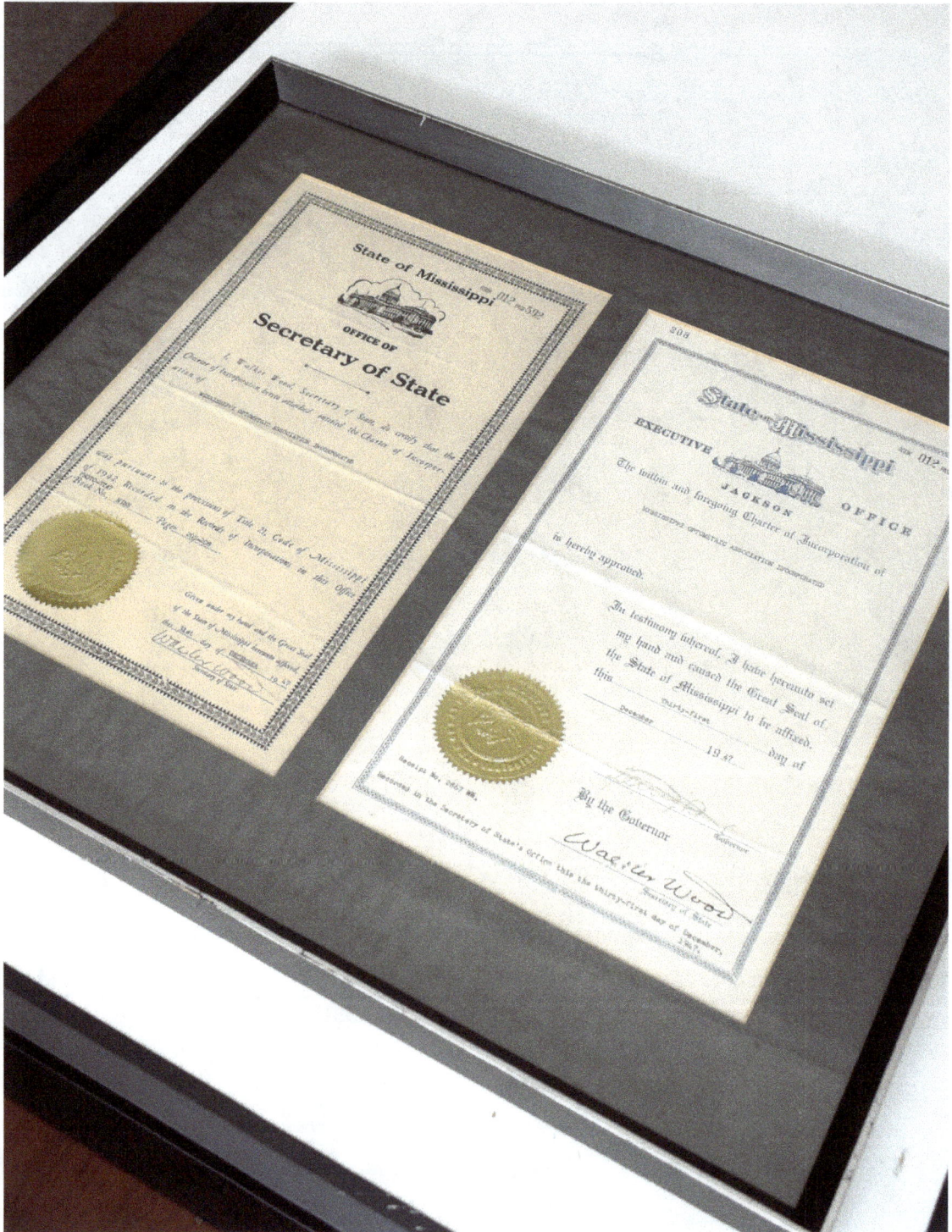

4. MOA Articles of Incorporation - 1947

PLAIN TALK

According to the present situation in Mississippi optometry today, it seems that we should take a positive stand on a few matters of importance to us all. This article expresses the personal feelings of the editor of the Mississippi Optometrist, who will be happy to print in the next issue any comments or differences of opinion you may have.

If you were able and/or interested enough to attend the 1950 MOA convention in Jackson, you know that the association passed a resolution regarding commercial practitioners. That resolution in its entirety is printed elsewhere in this issue.

A few optometrists have expressed their disapproval of this resolution. Some of them say it is absolutely necessary to retain their display windows, their neons, and commercial advertising. And the ones saying that have been in practice for a number of years, some for a good many years.

Optometry in Mississippi has come a long way since 1920. The older men are due our everlasting thanks for their labors in behalf of our profession. They are the ones who have built it to what it is today. However, should we be satisfied with the present or should we continue to build? Do you expect to drive a 1940 car in 1960?

What puzzles the editor is that the only ones expressing disapproval of the resolution are the very ones who would need to advertise least of all. We poor guys struggling in the first year or so of practice are the ones who certainly would be expected to need to advertise by displays and neons.

An optometrist who actually needs window displays and a lot of paid advertising after he has been practicing ten years is in pretty sad shape. He just doesn't have the stuff it takes to get there. I would hate to think that in five years I could not have enough patient-returns and patient-referrals to make a living.

For the few of you who think you need displays and neons, here are a few questions. Would you say that A. A. Schamber is a failure in optometry? He doesn't advertise by displays or neons. Johnny Price doesn't have to worry about his grocery bill. He doesn't advertise. Prospero De Marco's patients return to him and send their friends. He's one of the old timers who is keeping pace with the times. Patients drive hundreds of miles to get back to that grand old timer. M. L. Shannon, and his son, C. P., for glasses. There's just no substitute for professional ability and personality.

Brother, if you have to have a window display to get patients, there's something wrong with you as an optometrist. That's just plain talk and it may hit one or two. But for the few who have window displays now, it's just a habit. You can change that habit for a better one.

We are going to have an association in a few years second to none in our state. We can be proud to be known as a member of the Mississippi Optometric Association. It is my desire to be a member now and in the future and I expect to conduct myself and my practice in such a way as never to reflect on the prestige of my profession.

How do you feel about it? Am I right or wrong?

IRVIN MAULDIN, O.D., EDITOR
EDITORIAL - MISSISSIPPI OPTOMITRIST
APRIL 1950

5. Plain Talk Editorial, Mississippi Optometrist, 1950

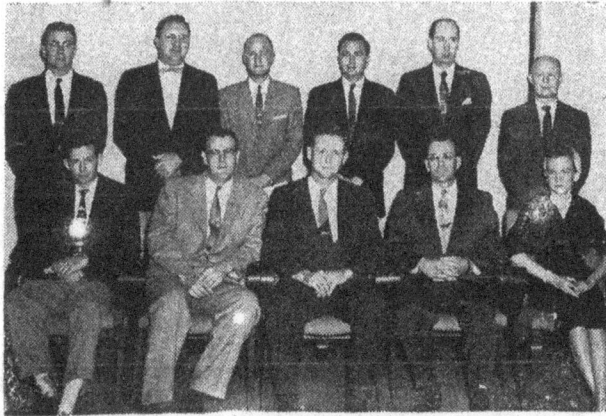

Above are shown the 1957 officers and directors of the Mississippi Optometric Association. Seated, left to right: Dr. Spurgeon Eure,, Hattiesburg, third vice-president; Dr. Walter Simpson, Booneville, second vice-president; Dr. Robert Griffin, Indianola, president; Dr. Ray Mitchell, Biloxi first vice-president; Dr. Nell Cochran, Kosciusko, director.

Standing are: left to right: Dr. Eric Muir, Cleveland, director; Dr. L. B. Adkins, Union, secretary-treasurer Dr. Sidney Watson, Kosciusko, fourth vice-president; Dr. Horace May, Newton, past president; Dr. William Hyde, Grenada, director and Dr. J. C. Reid, Holly Springs, director.

Optometric Greeting Card Available This Year

There IS simething new in cards for the holiday season—a greeting card designed especially for members of A. O. A. These cards are being produced for the Woman's Auxiliary to the A. O. A. and can be ordered through the state Auxiliaries which will benefit financially from the enterprise.

This is a handsome white greeting card with design and lettering in green. The message is suitable for all faiths. The Optometric Pledge is inscribed on the back and only members of A. O. A. are eligible to purchase them.

Use this greeting card for personal or professional lists. It can serve as a public relations mechanism and at the same time provide your Auxiliary with funds for Christmas projects. The latter are in themselves indirect public relations for optometry.

The cost is comparable to that charged for the most modest commercial greeting cards—they are boxed in sets of 25.

For more information contact Mrs. Horace May, president M. O. A. Auxiliary, Newton, Miss.

1958 MOA Membership Now Under Way

The 1958 membership campaign for the Mississippi Optometric Association is now under way, being led by Dr. Robert Griffin, Indianola, M. O. A. president.

Letters of information with forms indicating the desired method of paying the dues have been mailed out to all optometrists in the state. Dr. Griffin urges each one to complete the form and return it right away in order that plans for 1958 may be developed.

"The Mississippi Optometric Association affiliated with the American Optometric Association is working for you and for our profession," Dr. Griffin stated. "We must give them our support financially as well as with our actions if our progress is to continue."

Dr. Griffin pointed out the growth in Mississippi of the State Association over the past several years and the present high standards of practice over the state.

Next issue we start a new column on foods. Our first guest food editor will give his famous recipe for "stewed eggs."

6. 1957 MOA Officers

MISSISSIPPI OPTOMETRIC ASSOCIATION

ORGANIZATION

1960-1961

I. OFFICERS:

President: Dr. Frank Maier
President-Elect: Dr. W.M.Dickerson
Vice-President: Dr. Olin Mauldin
Administrative Director (Sec.-Treas.): Dr. Frank Houston
Board of Directors: Dr. William J. Goyer
                    Dr. Eric Muir
                    Dr. A.F. Hodges
                    Dr. Gene Felder
                    Dr. Paul Shannon
                    Dr. Walter Simpson (Immediate Past
                                        President)

II. EXECUTIVE COMMITTEES:

1. Interprofessional Relations Committee:

    M.O.A. President, President-Elect, Secretary, State
    Board President, Vice President, Secretary.

2. Legal and Legislative Watchdog Committee:

    Dr. H. A. Reese; Chairman, Dr. James Moye, Dr. Irvin
    Mauldin, Dr. Ray Mitchell.

3. Long-Term Planning Committee:

    Dr. Walter Simpson, Chairman
    Dr. Ray Mitchell
    Dr. Horace May
    Dr. Willard Commander
    Dr. James Moye
    Dr. H. A. Reese
    Pres., Pres.-Elect, Sec.-Treas.(Ex-offico)

4. Social and Health Care Trends Committee:
   (Vision Services Corp.)
    Dr. William J. Goyer, Chairman
    Dr. James Moye
    Dr. Spurgeon Eure

7. 1960 MOA Officers and Members (pg. 1)

5. Eye Care Commission:

    Dr. Rayford N. Edgar, Chairman
    Dr. Irvin Mauldin
    Dr. R. B. Griffin
    Dr. Ray Mitchell

6. Liason Officer for M.O.A. Auxiliary:

    Dr. W.M. Dickerson

7. General Attorney: Richard A. Billups, Jr., Esq.

8. Editor, "MISSISSIPPI OPTOMETRIST", Dr. M. I. Mauldin

9. O.E.P. State Director: Dr. Armin von Seutter

III. Department of Public Information:

    Dr. Paul Shannon, Director

Speakers Bureau: Dr. Nell Cochran, Director

IV. Department of Education:

    Dr. Eric Muir, Director

1. Contact Lens Committee
    Dr. L. O. Embrey, Jr., Chairman
    Dr. Ray F. Mitchell
    Dr. Fred Smith
    Dr. Spurgeon Eure
    Dr. Frank Edgar
    Dr. Eric Muir (Director Consultant)

2. Visual Training and Developmental Vision Committee:
    (AOA- Visual Problems in Children & Youth Comm.)
    Dr. Armin von Seutter, Chairman
    Dr. A. F. Hodges
    Dr. T. M. Pierce
    Dr. William J. Goyer (Director Consultant)

3. Practice Management Committee:
    Dr. James Moye, Chairman
    Dr. W.F. Clark
    Dr. Horace May
    Dr. Paul Shannon (Director Consultant)

7. 1960 MOA Officers and Members (pg. 2)

4. Visual Problems of the Aging & Subnormal Vision Aids

Committee :
Dr. Walter Simpson, Chairman
Dr. S. W. Hora
Dr. James E. Gooch
Dr. Armin von Seutter
Dr. Paul Lycette
Dr. Eric Muir
Dr. Gene Felder (Director Consultant)

5. Research & Standards Committee:
Dr. Sidney Watson, Chairman
Dr. H. A. Reese
Dr. Armin von Seutter
Dr. Paul Shannon (Director Consultant)

V. Department of Organization:
Dr. W. M. Dickerson, Director

1. Vocational Guidance & Scholarship Committee:
Dr. Robert B. Griffin, Chairman
Dr. Rayford Edgar
Dr. W. S. (Billy) Harper
Dr. James Houston
Dr. Frank Houston (Executive Consultant)

2. Assistance to Graduates & Undergraduates Committee:
Dr. A. F. Hodges, Chairman
Dr. C. P. Tillman
Dr. J. R. Lamb
Dr. Frank Houston, (Executive Consultant)

3. Insurance & Tax Advisory Committee:
Dr. Ray Mitchell, Chairman
Mr. Richard A. Billups, Fr. (Legal Consultant)
Dr. William J. Goyer (Director Consultant)
Dr. Frank Houston (Executive Consultant)

4. Ethics (Rules of Practice) Committee:
Dr. Horace May, Chairman
Dr. Paul Lycette
Dr. J. K. Suttle
Dr. L. B. Adkins
Dr. W. F. Clark
Dr. A. F. Hodges (Director Consultant)

5. American Optometric Foundation Committee:
Dr. H. A. Reese, Chairman
Dr. Eric Muir
Dr. Nash Cochran

7. 1960 MOA Officers and Members (pg. 3)

103

VI. Department of Public Services:
        Dr. Olin Mauldin, Director

    1. Motorist's Vision Committee:
        Dr. Gene Felder, Chairman(Jackson Group)
        Dr. H. A. Reese   Dr. Paul Lycette
        Dr. Richard Cortese   Dr. John I. Magee
        Dr. Olin Mauldin   Dr. Robert H. Marsh
        Dr. A. B. Crane   Dr. Evelyn Watson
        Dr. Jim Wright   Dr. Curtis B. Magee
        Dr. Roland Stevens   Dr. Harry Watson

    2. Fair Booth Committee:
        Dr. Gene Felder, Chairman
        (Jackson Group)   (State at large)
        Dr. Paul Lycett   Dr. H. A. Reese
        Dr. John I. Magee   Dr. Richard Cortese
        Dr. Curtis B. Magee   Dr. Olin Mauldin
        Dr. Robert H. Marsh   Dr. A. B. Crane
        Dr. Harry Watson   Dr. Jim Wright
        Dr. Evelyn Watson   Dr. Roland Stevens

    3. Occupational Vision Committee:
        Dr. W. M. Dickerson, Chairman
        Dr. Robert Mitchell
        Dr. Harlan Sears
        Dr. Avery McKinley
        Dr. T. M. Pierce
        Dr. Olin Mauldin (Director Consultant)

    4. Liason With Lions Sight Service Committee:
        Dr. Avery McKinley, Chairman
        Dr. Bolivar A. Sims
        Dr. James L. Houston
        Dr. James Gooch
        Dr. Paul Shannon (Director Consultant)

    5. Civil Defense & Military Optometry Committee:
        Dr. Harry Watson, Chairman
        Dr. Walter Simpson
        Dr. William Starr
        Dr. F. B. Maier (Executive Consultant)

VII. Mississippi State Board of Optometry
        Dr. M. I. Mauldin, President
            Corinth, Mississippi
        Dr. W. E. Clark, Secretary
            Meridian, Mississippi
        Dr. James M. Moye
            Laurel, Mississippi
        Dr. Rayford N. Edgar
            Water Valley, Mississippi
        Dr. H. A. Reese
            Cleveland, Mississippi

7. 1960 MOA Officers and Members (pg. 4)

MISSISSIPPI OPTOMETRIC ASSOCIATION

AUGUST 20, 1960

1. L. B. Adkins, Union
2. D. H. Adler, 110 Southern
    Bldg., Meridian
3. B. F. Bleuer, 131 Canal St.
    Picayune
4. J. M. Bleuer, 210 Howard Ave.
    Biloxi
5. James E. Byrd, 1822 25th Ave.,
    Gulfport
6. Norman Campbell, Senatobia
7. W. F. Clark, Dixie Towers Bldg.
    Meridian
8. Nash Cochran, Cleveland
9. Nell Cochran, Kosciusko
10. W. M. Commander, John B.
    Perkins Bldg., Brookhaven
11. A. R. Cortese, Crystal Springs
12. A. B. Crane, P.O. Box 208
    Pascagoula
13. W. H. Dearman, Saenger Bldg.,
    Hattiesburg
14. W. M. Dickerson, 309 Main St.,
    Tupelo
15. Paul A. Doherty, 606 Franklin
    St. Natchez
16. Frank R. Edgar, Short St.,
    Hattiesburg
17. J. H. Edgar, Short Street,
    Hattiesburg
18. Rayford N. Edgar, Water Valley
19. L. O. Embrey, Jr. 314 N.
    Magnolia, Laurel
20. S. B. Euro, 2011 Mamie St.,
    Hattiesburg
21. Joseph F. Fasold, 1219, 24th
    Ave., Gulfport
22. Gene W. Felder, Mart 51,
    Jackson
23. James E. Gooch, 324 Main St.
    Columbus
24. William J. Goyer, Carter Bldg.
    Hattiesburg
25. James B. Grace, Canton
26. R. B. Griffin, Indianola
27. Ted Harden, P. O. Box 126,
    Columbus
28. Lauren Harper, 1st Nt. Bank,
    Bldg., Laurel
29. W. S. Harper, Jr., Batesville
30. Frank Headley, Port Gibson
31. A. F. Hodges, Amory
32. James F. Hogg, Arcade Bldg.
    Greenville
33. John J. Hora, Corinth
34. S. W. Hora, Jr. Corinth
35. F. E. Houston, Lexington
36. James L. Houston, Belzoni
37. James C. Hinman, 424 Jackson
    Ave., Pascagoula
38. William T. Hyde, Grenada
39. M. H. Jacobs, P.O. Box 432
    Pascagoula
40. William R. Keller, Pinehurst
    Hotel Bldg., Laurel
41. Alvin M. Labens, 13 Third St.
    Clarksdale
42. J. R. Lamb, Dispatch Bldg.,
    Columbus
43. Ned Lewis, P.O. Box 1122,
    Laurel
44. A. E. Lorance, Jr., 1213
    Washington St., Vicksburg
45. Paul W. Lycette, 240 Meadow
    Brook Rd. Jackson
46. Curtis B. Magee, 214 N.
    Congress, Jackson
47. John I. Magee, P.O. Box 6686
    Jackson 4
48. Frank B. Maier, Aberdeen
49. R. H. Marsh, 104 W. Capitol
    St. Jackson
50. G. R. Martindale, Ripley
51. Irvin Mauldin, Corinth
52. Olin B. Mauldin, McComb
53. Horace L. May, Newton
54. Charles W. Maxey, Charleston
55. Ray F. Mitchell, P.O. Drawer
    268, Biloxi
56. Robert J. Mitchell, Moss Point
57. James M. Moye, P. O. Box 1122
    Laurel
58. Wiley H. Mock, Leyeser Bldg.
    Greenville

7. 1960 MOA Officers and Members (pg. 5)

59. M. E. Muir, Cleveland
60. A. H. McKinley, 110 N. Commerce St., Natchez
61. Carlton McMillan, Carthage
62. W. D. Newsom, Waynesboro
63. T. M. Pierce, Amory
64. John E. Price, Booneville
65. H. A. Reese, Cleveland
66. W. P. Reese, 246 Washington Ave. Greenville
67. J. F. Rhodes, Ackerman
68. David L. Rogers, Drew
69. J. W. Rothchild, Oxford
70. W. C. Russo, Bay St. Louis
71. Claude S. Sarphie, 509 Main St., Hattiesburg
72. H.H. Sears, West Point
73. Paul K. Shannon, New Albany
74. Robert L. Shannon, Pontotoc
75. R. L. Shannon, New Albany
76. W. C. Simpson, Booneville
77. B. A. Sims, 416 Howard St. Greenwood
78. Fred W. Smith, Jr., Brookhaven
79. W. H. Starr, 1309 26th Ave., Gulfport
80. R. G. Stribling, Philadelphia
81. R. H. Stevens, Yazoo City
82. Joe K. Suttle, Louisville
83. James T. Thomas, Yazoo City
84. S. W. Thorne, Hazelhurst
85. Charles P. Tillman, Houston
86. Armin von Seutter, Starkville
87. Carl R. von Seutter, Canton
88. Lester L. Walraven, Louisville
89. Evelyn Watson, 2519 W. Capitol St. Jackson
90. Harry Watson, 107 N. President St. Jackson
91. Sidney J. Watson, Kosciusko
92. Frank Weinberg, McComb
93. William A. Williamson, 533 Washington Ave, Greenville
94. James E. Wright, Forest

NON-MEMBER OPTOMETRISTS

1. R. D. Burns, West Point
2. T. P. Cote, Sr., 145 E. Capitol St., Jackson
3. T. P. Cote, Jr. 104 W. Capitol St., Jackson
4. V. L. Coumar, P.O. Box 909, Gulfport
5. S. D. Douglas, Bacot Bldg., Pascagoula
6. Jesse Griffin, Starkville
7. M. Harrison, 1200 22th Ave. Meridian
8. S. E. Lawrence, Columbia
9. R. I. Lopez, 117 W. Capitol St. Jackson
10. Nettie M. Loper, Greenwood
11. M. S. Melvin, 117 W. Capitol St. Jackson
12. G. D. Mitchell, Picayune
13. Chris C. Muir, Winona
14. J. H. McCloskey, Philadelphia
15. D. H. Orkin, 204 W. Capitol, Jackson
16. W. B. Owen, Starkville
17. J. L. Rothchild, College Hill Rd. Oxford
18. A. A. Schamber, Dixie Towers Bldg., Meridian
19. G. E. Seal, Tylertown
20. C. P. Shannon, Pontotoc
21. Homer Skinner, Philadelphia
22. A. N. Wilson, Tupelo
23. J. K. Worley, Yazoo City

7. 1960 MOA Officers and Members (pg. 6)

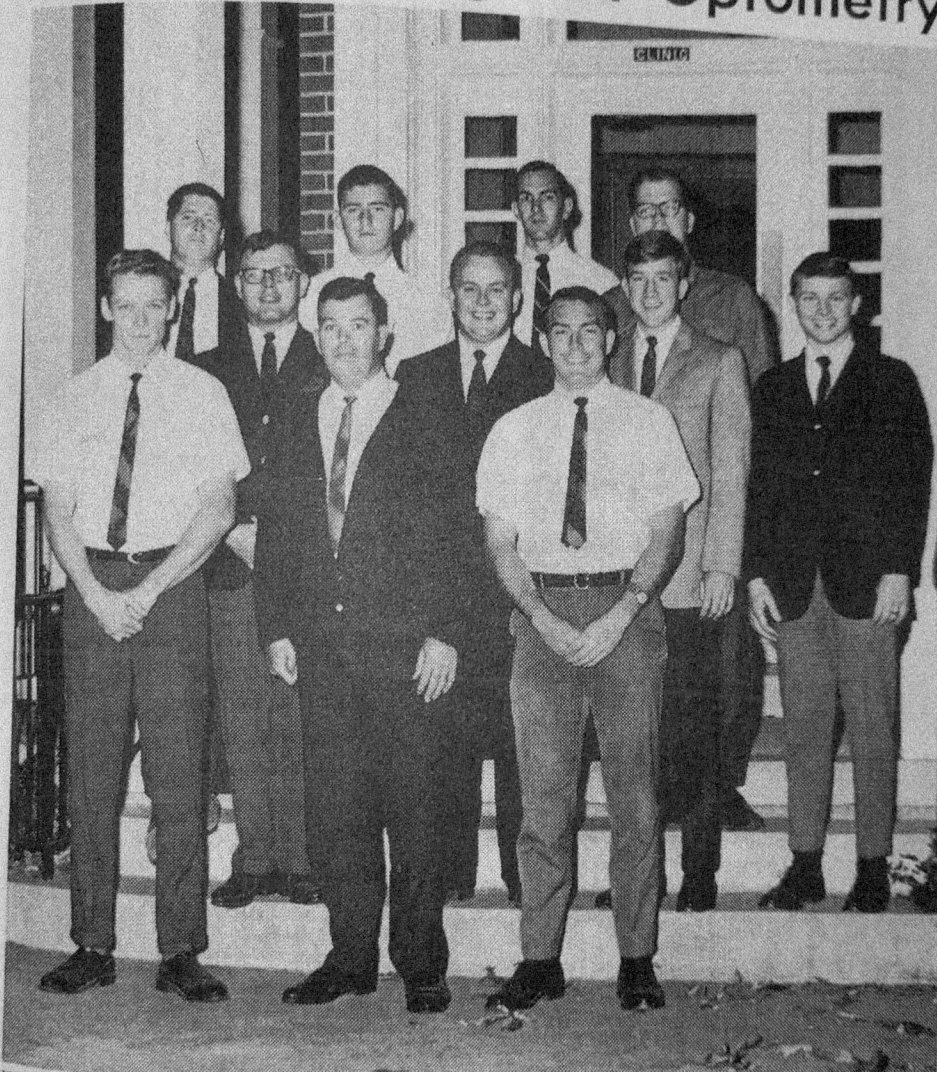

The Mississippi Optometrist

Page 5

1967 Mississippi Club
Southern College Of Optometry

Front row, l to r: Bernard Ellis, Cleveland, senior; Charles Ingram, Memphis, senior; Watts Davis, Laurel, senior; Second row: W. C. Maples, Hattiesburg, junior; James Coe, Memphis, junior, class secretary; Bill Cochran, Kosciusko, junior, class president; Earl Malone, McComb, junior. Third row: Bob Montgomery, Southhaven, junior; Kelly Durham, Grenada, sophomore; Bob Carty, Indianola, sophomore, class vice-president; Paul Clark, Magee, sophomore.

8. SCO Mississippi Club, 1967

Children Activities

<u>Sunday, June 3</u>

T.V. Room - Biloxi Room

3:30 Trip to Deer Ranch

6:00 Meal at McDonalds

<u>Monday, June 4</u>

T.V. Room - Biloxi Room

3:00 Gulf Hills Dude Ranch

5:30 Hamburger Party - Boston Room

7:00 Movies

<u>Tuesday, June 5</u>

T.V. Room - Biloxi Room

10:00 Goofy Golf & Amusement Park

Baby Sitters Available at all times
Biloxi Room

1973

Mississippi Optometric Association

Convention

Sheraton - Biloxi Motor Inn

Sunday - June 3

9:00 am Registration - Coffee and donuts courtesy
of Optometric Auxiliary - Lobby

10:00 am Preconvention Meeting - Officers and
Board of Directors - Boston Room

11:00 am Church (see Hotel Directory)

1:30 pm Convention Opening - Gulf Room C
Invocation - Brother Jim Bowers
Welcome Address - Frank Barhanovich
Commissioner
Response - Dr. Roland Stevens,
President of MOA

2:00 pm Continuing Education Course - Gulf Room A
Developmental & Perceptual training -
Dr. Rod Fields, W.C. Maples, & Howard Jenkins
& Max Edrington
How to Work Effectively with Your State
Legislature - Dr. Billy Cochran
Contact Lens Fitting - Dr. Wayne Bensman

Continuing Education Course - Gulf Room D
How to increase your Optometric Practice
by $20,000.00 - Dr. Joyce Adema

4:00 pm Past and Present Auxiliary Officers
Meeting - Jackson Room

5:00 pm MOA Auxiliary Meeting - Jackson Room
MOA General Business Session - Gulf Room A

6:30 pm HOSPITALITY - Rooms

7:30 pm Seafood Jamboree - Pool Patio
Entertainment - Bob & Patti Ryan

9:00 pm Night Life - Fiesta

Monday - June 4

7:00 am Golf Tournament - Shopping, etc. for the
ladies

12:00 pm Auxiliary Luncheon - Top of Sheraton
Dr. Joyce Adema - Thursdays Child

2:00 pm Continuing Education Course - North Room
Analytical Observations and Interpreta-
tions - Dr. George Slade

4:00 pm MOA General Business Session - North Room
Tea - In Honor of Mrs. Mark Forgues
National Auxiliary President

5:00 pm HOSPITALITY - Rooms

7:00 pm Cocktail Hour - Gulf Rooms A and B

8:00 pm Banquet - East Ball Room
Master of Ceremony - Dr. Billy Cochran
Guest Speaker - Dr. Spurqueon Eure
SCO President
Band - Personalities

Tuesday - June 5

6:00 am Fishing Trip - Silver Dollar

9:00 am Continuing Education Course - Gulf Room A
Analytical Observations of Visual
Performance and Development - Dr. George
Slade

10:00 am Brunch and Fashion Show - Top of Sheraton
Guest Speaker - Mrs. Mark Forgues

9. MOA Annual Convention Program, 1973

108

FOCUS

Strategic Planning Retreat
Lake Tiak O'Khata

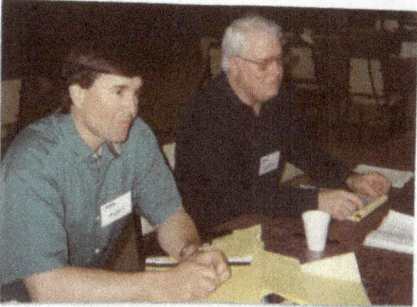

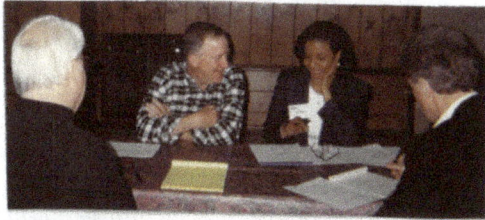

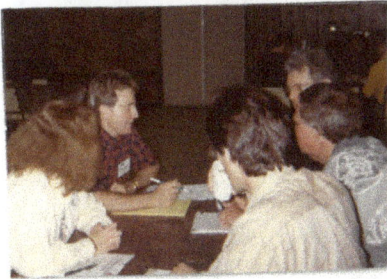

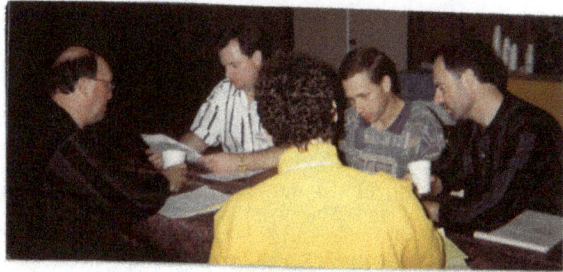

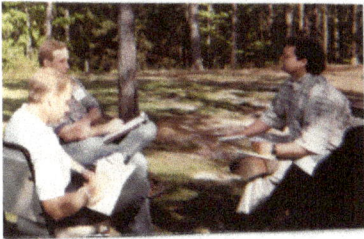

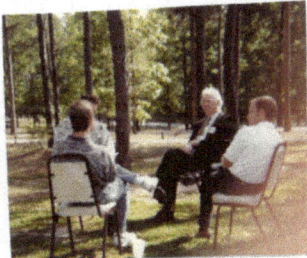

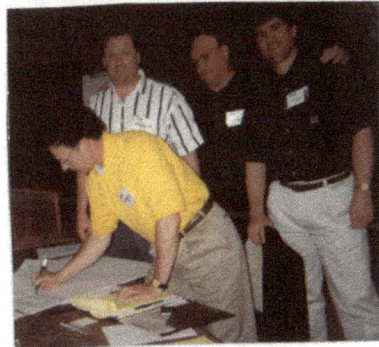

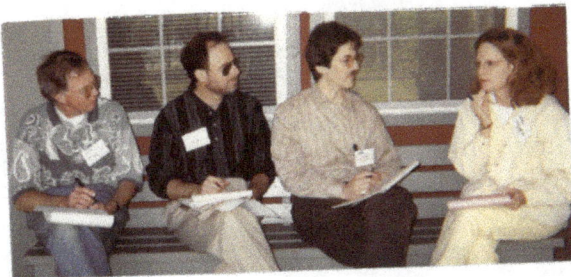

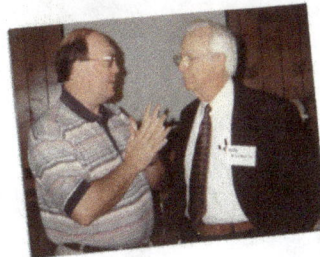

10. Photos from 1981 Strategic Planning Session, 1981

10/27/2020   Mail - Cochran, William - Outlook

PRESIDENT'S MESSAGE

The greatest reward that Mississippi Doctors of Optometry have received for their use of pharmaceuticals these past three years is the high level of quality optometric care provided the public and the recognition of that care by our State Legislature. We have been told that the two most highly contested pieces of legislation this season were teachers salaries and the optometry bill. That gives us some perspective of the attack the medical lobby leveled at us. Even with their megabucks medical association, multiple lobbyists and intensive misrepresentation of facts -- optometry's quality of care for the public prevailed.

James P. Brownlee, O.D.,
President

The credit for this success in communication of the truth lies in the dedication of those who want to see the public served best. Our gratitude must be extended to our legislative advocate and advisor Clifford Thompson for his expertise and experience, and for his character in confronting the formidable medical lobby, to Helen St. Clair for her astute organizational skills and seemingly inexhaustible energy and confidence in our ability to succeed, to our legislative chairman Larry Routt for his time, talent and tremendous effort in moving us toward our goals, to our LGA committee members Eric Muir, Jack Hora, and Jeff Minor for their experience guidance and hours of work, to our district chairman and co-workers B.A. Sims, Danny Clifton, Gene Felder, Glen Stribling, Glenn Cochran, Carl Von Seutter, Mike Quint and Sallye Sawyer for critical communications at the grass roots level, to the very special esteem in which Senator John White is held by his legislative peers, to irreplaceable contributions by Jerry Hayes, Max Edrington and Avery McKinley, and to each and every Mississippi doctor of optometry who worked to strengthen the quality primary care provided our patients.

Our congratulations go out to you for "Making It Happen".

GOVERNOR BILL ALLAIN SIGNS SB 2796

On March 22nd, Governor Bill Allain signed SB 2796. Now, Mississippi optometrists have a concrete law that allows utilization of diagnostic pharmaceuticals. The Bill does not have any adverse amendments. It is exactly like the present law except the repealer is removed.

The Bill passed the House on March 12th by a vote of 98-16, following the removal of amendments. Mississippi optometrists are to be commended for individual efforts during this legislative session.

Several members have inquired about the 1982 vote in the House of Representatives on HB 475. It was 93-25.

-1-

11. President's Message, Dr. Jim Brownlee, 1982

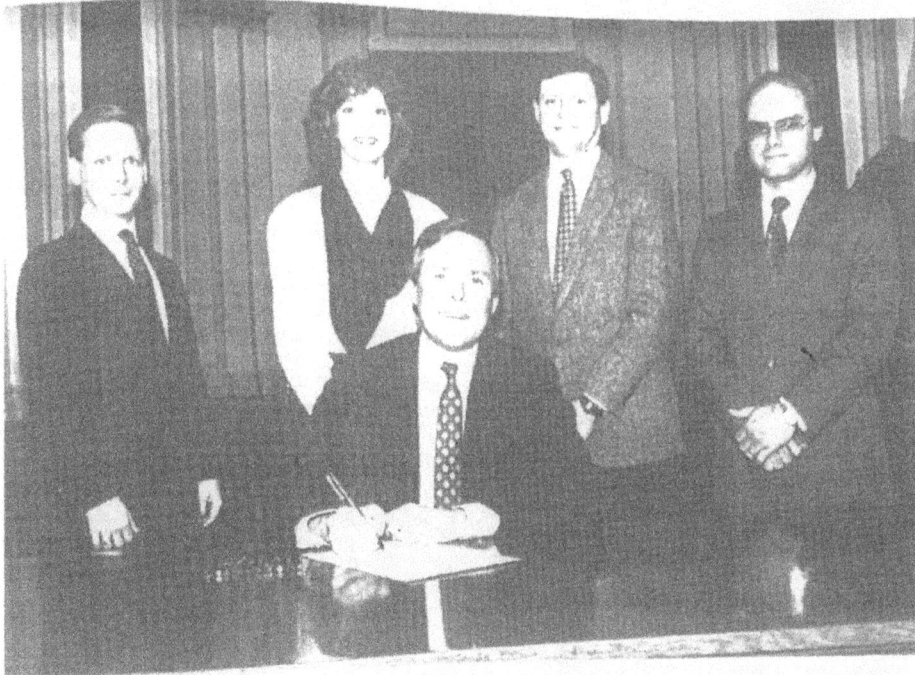

"OPTOMETRISTS WITH A HEART"
VISION USA/MISSISSIPPI PROJECT

Governor Ray Mabus is pictured signing a proclamation for 1989 Save Your Vision Week in Mississippi. Pictured from left to right are: Glen H. Stribling, O.D., Crystal Springs; Ann A. Williams, O.D., Hattiesburg; W. Boyce Craig, O.D., Canton and Ridgeland and C. Chris Collins, O.D., Vicksburg. Dr. Craig is Save Your Vision Week/Month Chairman.

12. Save Your Vision Week, Proclamation, 1989

MISSISSIPPI BOARD OF OPTOMETRY NEWS

Volume 5 Issue 1	April 2005

BOARD MEMBERS

The following is a list of the members of the Board currently serving the congressional districts in our state:
Fred Mothershed, O.D.
E. Watts Davis, O.D.
Lowell Jones, O.D.
Charles Barnes, O.D.
W. Gil Davis, O.D.

BOARD MEETINGS

Tentative schedule for 2005:
January 8th
July 9th
November – MOA
Additional meeting may be held as such times and places that the Board shall determine.

BOARD LICENSED OPTOMETRISTS

The Board would like to offer their congratulations to the following optometrists who were licensed on January 2005.
Terri Shannon, O.D.
Carrie Gautreau, O.D.
Bhavani Yedulapuram, O.D.
Heather Borgon, O.D.

UPCOMING EVENTS

The Mississippi Optometric Association Convention will be held at the Island House Hotel in Orange Beach, AL on June 17-19, 2005.
The 86th annual ARBO meeting will be in Dallas, Texas at the Gaylord Texan Resort & Convention Center on June 19-21, 2005.
The AOA Annual Congress will follow on

SENATE BILL 2682, ORAL MEDICATION CONTINUING EDUCATION

Governor Haley Barbour has signed Senate Bill 2682 and the effective date of the legislation is July 1, 2005. At a Board meeting immediately following the signing, the board voted to require all active, therapeutically certified Optometrists licensed in Mississippi to attend a review course regarding the administration of oral medications. This course will be **mandatory.**
All Optometrists that this will affect will be mailed details as they become available.

ANNOUNCMENTS

There will be a reception to honor Ms. Helen St. Clair during the June Mississippi Optometric Association Convention. Ms. St Clair has announced her plans to retire as the executive Director of the MOA. Her tireless efforts, hard work, sincere concern, and years of dedication have been greatly appreciated by the State Board. She will be sorely missed.

Rule 12.5

Rule 12.5 requires all Optometrists to obtain their Therapeutic certification by December 2006. Pennsylvania College of Optometry will be offering a 100 hours Ocular Therapeutics course on June 5-15, 2005. The cost will be $2775.00. For more information, contact Jennifer Lau at the Center for Continuing Education at PCO at

13. Senate Bill 2682, Oral Medication Bill

1948 – 1950	William J. Goyer, O.D.	1989 – 1990	Danny Ray Clifton, O.D.
1950 – March	M. Eric Muir, O.D.	1990 – 1991	Glenn M. Cochran, O.D.
1950 – 1952 Sept.	H. Andy Reese, O.D.	1991 – 1992	Ann A. Williams, O.D.
1952 – March	John E. Price, O.D.	1992 – 1993	William M. Dickerson, Jr., O.D.
1953 – 1954	Willard M. Commander, O.D.	1993 – 1994	Glen Hanson Stribling, O.D.
1954 – 1956	James M. Moye, O.D.	1994 – 1995	Mark W. Martindale, O.D.
1956 – 1957	Horace L. May, O.D.	1995 – 1996	Frank Evans, Jr., O.D.
1957 – 1958	R. B. Griffin, O.D.	1996 – 1997	Michael F. Quint, O.D.
1958 – 1959	Ray F. Mitchell, O.D.	1997 – 1998	Glen H. Stone, O.D.
1959 – 1960	Walter C. Simpson, O.D.	1998 – 1999	Frank Reese, O.D.
1960 – 1961	Frank B. Maier, Jr., O.D.	1999 – 2000	R. Kent Stribling, O.D.
1961 – 1962	William M. Dickerson, Sr., O.D.	2000 – 2001	William Gil Davis, O.D.
1962 – 1964	Arnold Fred Hodges, O.D.	2001 – 2002	William M. E. Strickland, O.D.
1964 – 1965	Lois Bernell Adkins, O.D.	2002 – 2003	Wilburn Lord, Jr., O.D.
1965 – 1966	W. H. Starr, O.D.	2003 – 2004	Linda D. Johnson, O.D.
1966 – 1967	Richard G. Stribling, O.D.	2004 – 2005	David H. Curtis, O.D.
1967 – 1968	Paul W. Lycette, O.D.	2005 – 2006	Craig Belk, O.D.
1968 – 1969	Billy G. Lightsey, O.D.	2006 – 2007	Amy Crigler, O.D.
1969 – 1970	Fred G. Blevins, O.D.	2007 – 2008	Steven Reed, O.D.
1970 – 1972	John H. Mohr, O.D.	2008 – 2009	David L. Parker, O.D.
1972 – 1973	Roland H. Stevens, O.D.	2009 – 2010	Susanne Cunningham, O.D.
1973 – 1974	Charlie Collins, O.D.	2010 – 2011	Philip Marler, O.D.
1974 – 1976	James E. Herrington, O.D.	2011 – 2012	Reggie Dampier, O.D.
1976 – 1977	John R. White, O.D.	2012 – 2013	Bradley Thompson, O.D.
1977 – 1978	W. E. (Billy) Cochran, O.D.	2013 – 2014	Eric Randle, O.D.
1978 – 1979	Travis M. Pierce, O.D.	2014 – 2015	Nicole Monroe, O.D.
1979 – 1980	E. Watts Davis, O.D.	2015 – 2016	Greg Loose, O.D.
1980 – 1981	William W. Stanfill, O.D.	2016 – 2017	Mike Weeden, O.D.
1981 – 1983	Robert G. Traylor, O.D.	2017 – Jul 2018	Tonyatta Hairston, O.D.
1983 – 1984	George R. Martindale, O.D.	Jul 2018 – 2019	Amy Crigler, O.D.
1984 – 1985	James P. Brownlee, O.D.	2019 – 2020	Jason "Bo" Beddingfield, O.D.
1985 – 1986	Joseph J. Joseph, O.D.	2020 – 2021	Dax Eckard, O.D.
1986 – 1987	Thomas G. Hollis, O.D.		
1987 – 1988	William Earl Malone, O.D.		
1988 – 1989	Charles Lowell Jones, O.D.		

14. Past Presidents of the Mississippi Optometric Association

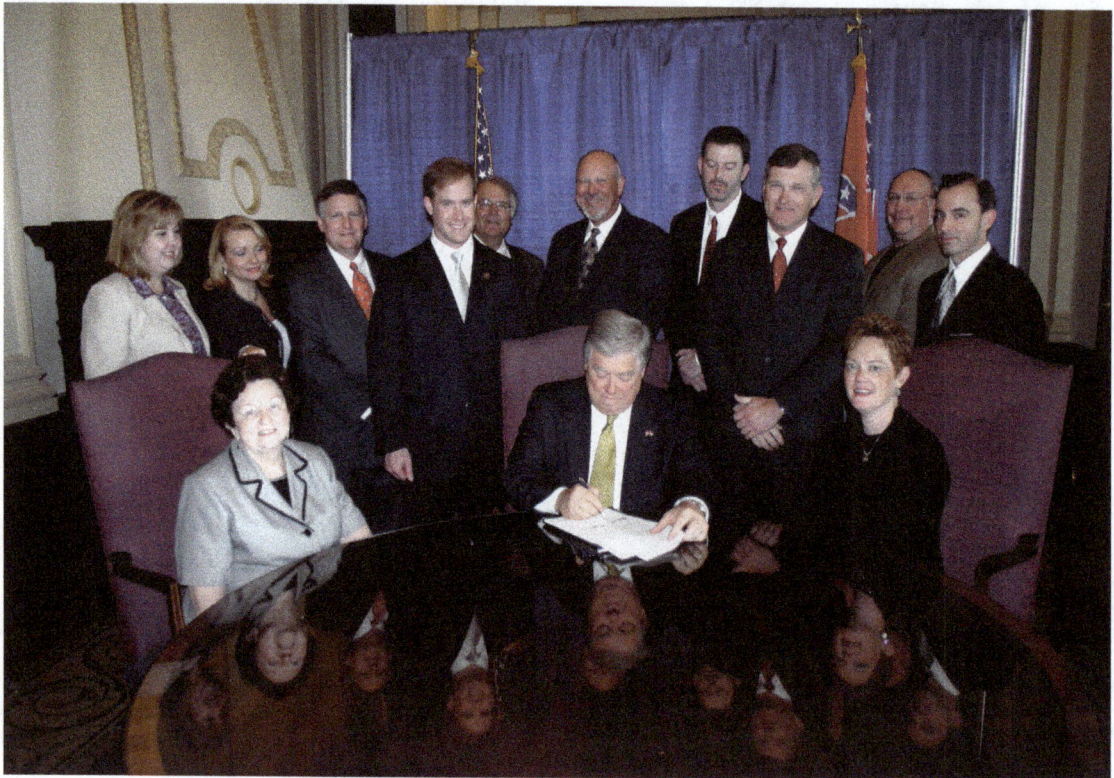

15. Photo of SB 2682 being signed, 2005

Front row, L-R: Helen St. Clair, CAE, Governor Haley Barbour, Dr. Amy Crigler. Back row, L-R: Lee Ann Mayo, Clare Hester, Dr. Fred Mothershed, Dr. David Cheatham, unknown, Dr. C. Lowell Jones, Dr. Chuck Barnes, Dr. David Curtis, Dr. Watts Davis, Dr. Chris Evans.

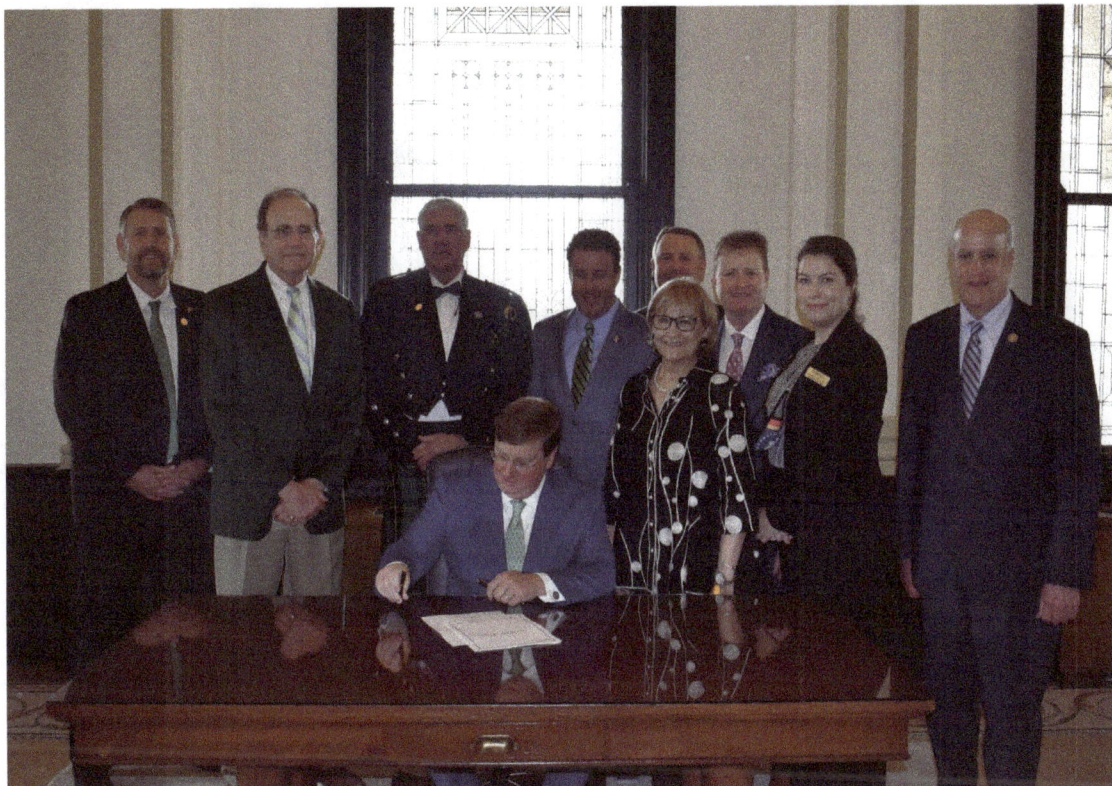

16. Photo of HB 1302 being signed, 2021

L-R: Senator Chris Caughman, Lt. Gov. Delbert Hosemann, Senator Kevin Blackwell, Senator David Parker, OD, Speaker Pro Tem Jason White, Dr. Dax Eckard, Sarah E. Link, CAE, Representative Scott Bounds. Front: Gov. Tate Reeves, Linda Ross Aldy, CAE

www.ingramcontent.com/pod-product-compliance
Lightning Source LLC
Chambersburg PA
CBHW061958090426
42811CB00006B/982

* 9 7 8 0 5 7 8 9 8 1 1 5 4 *